CHICKEN UNGA FEVER

WHITAKER is a writer and practising doctor.
s 'Health Matters' column appears fortnightly
the *New Statesman*. As well as his writing on
lical matters, he is the award-winning author of
novels, most recently *Sister Sebastian's Library*
ₒ₁₆) and *You* (2018), both published by Salt.

ALSO BY PHIL WHITAKER

Eclipse of the Sun (1997)
Triangulation (1999)
The Face (2002)
Freak of Nature (2007)
Sister Sebastian's Library (2016)
You (2018)

DR PHIL WHITAKER

CHICKEN UNGA FEVER

Stories from the medical frontline

CROMER

PUBLISHED BY SALT PUBLISHING 2018

2 4 6 8 10 9 7 5 3 1

First published in Great Britain in 2018 by
Salt Publishing Ltd
12 Norwich Road, Cromer, Norfolk NR27 0AX United Kingdom

www.saltpublishing.com

Salt Publishing Limited Reg. No. 5293401

A CIP catalogue record for this book is available from the British Library

ISBN 978 1 78463 154 3 (Paperback edition)
ISBN 978 1 78463 155 0 (Electronic edition)

Typeset in Neacademia by Salt Publishing

Printed and bound in Great Britain by Clays Ltd, Elcograf S.p.A

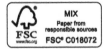

For my sister, Sue, and my brother, Mike

The articles in this collection first appeared as 'Health Matters' columns in the *New Statesman*, and are reproduced with kind permission. I am very grateful to the editor, Jason Cowley, for commissioning the column back in 2013, and to the arts editor, Kate Mossman, for shepherding the column over the ensuing five years with good humour and an unfailingly keen editorial eye.

CONTENTS

MUSINGS

IN HOURS

OFF DUTY

IN HOURS

BUZZERS AND MEETERS

GPs CAN BE divided into two distinct groups: 'buzzers' and 'meeters'. The former stay put in their consulting rooms, employing a variety of devices such as buzzers or intercoms to call their patients through. 'Meeters', on the other hand, walk along to collect each patient from the waiting room in person.

We are 'meeters' in my practice. I like the brief interlude of physical activity, which helps clear the mind in readiness for the next consultation. Equally important is the opportunity to begin putting patients at ease, greeting them with a smile and making small talk as we walk the corridor together. The rapport-building helps the consultation get off to a good start, rather than the patient arriving 'cold' at my consulting room door.

'Meeting' also provides valuable advance information. Musculoskeletal problems are the most obvious: back pain is instantly recognisable from the way someone gets out of their chair. Hip, knee, and ankle pathology produce characteristic gaits. The severity of respiratory problems can be gauged by the degree of breathlessness with exertion. Eye contact, body posture, and facial expression when crossing the waiting room give clues as to the patient's state of mind - depression, acute anxiety, or frustration and anger all transmit themselves clearly, and one can prepare oneself for the likely tenor of the consultation.

'Waiting room diagnoses' are sometimes memorable, as in the case of Simon, a 45-year-old I went to collect a little while ago. His notes had already revealed him to be an infrequent attender, making it more likely that he would be coming about something significant. When I called his name, his wife got up to accompany him – often a sign of high levels of concern; sometimes indicative of a reluctant male being frogmarched to the doctor by a spouse who's decided enough-is-enough. Both their faces were taut with worry. By the time Simon reached me I had the full picture. He was noticeably out of breath after walking just those dozen yards. A glance told me the reason: he was strikingly pale, a sign of gross anaemia. The amount of the oxygen-carrying red pigment (haemoglobin) in his blood was very low.

As we made our way along the corridor, I thought ahead. There are several types of anaemia, but by far the commonest is iron-deficiency. This arises either because of inadequate iron in the diet (rare in the UK), failure to absorb iron from food (coeliac disease is the most frequent culprit), or – most often – sustained loss of blood. Women of reproductive age quite commonly become anaemic from excessive menstrual bleeding. In a male of Simon's age, however, a marked iron-deficiency anaemia is unusual and worrying – it is a typical presentation of gastrointestinal cancer, an otherwise unsuspected tumour leaking small amounts of blood into the bowel day after day until haemoglobin levels fall sufficient to cause symptoms. By the time Simon, his wife, and I had seated ourselves in my consulting room, I was braced for a delicate discussion. And once Simon had admitted that he'd been keeping quiet about periodic blood in his stools for some months, the path ahead was clear.

Since 2000, GPs have been able to refer suspected cancer cases under the 'two week wait' (2WW) rule, ensuring that investigations are undertaken speedily. The only proviso is the patient must be made aware that cancer is a distinct possibility, both to ensure they attend the urgent appointment slot and to prepare the ground for any discussion that may be needed at the hospital. In Simon's case, he required direct inspection of his lower digestive tract. Colonoscopy is a fairly unpleasant procedure, not least because endoscopic inspection of the lower bowel is only possible after a purge with powerful laxatives. Simon was going to have to spend a couple of days staying very close to a loo.

There was a lot to explain and prepare him for, not least the fact that, were a bowel cancer to be discovered, there was a reasonable prospect of cure. Survival rates in the UK have more than doubled over the past thirty years, with at least half of patients being disease-free after ten years, rising to a 90% cure rate if the tumour is detected at an early stage. Even though the outlook is far from gloomy, and even though the 2WW rule has dramatically shortened the time spent in limbo waiting for results, the uncertainty can be very difficult to cope with. Simon and his wife were understandably anxious, but I was impressed by the phlegmatic way in which they greeted each new piece of information, all the more so because they have a young family. Simon's comments stayed with me: about how they would remain calm, and square up to whatever they needed to deal with.

A couple of weeks later, a fax brought the good news: Simon was clear of cancer. The bleeding was from an unusual blood vessel anomaly in the bowel wall, readily treatable by laser. He and his wife made an appointment a few days later to discuss the next steps. It was a genuine pleasure to see the smiles on their faces as they came across the waiting room towards me, a sight I would have missed were I a 'buzzer' rather than a 'greeter'.

BITES

E RICA WAS AT the end of her tether. 'I've had the council round several times, they've fumigated the whole place twice, and still I'm getting bitten.'

I peered at her lower legs. There were scattered red lumps, and lots of scratch marks. The environmental health department's pest control officer, having exhausted his insecticidal repertoire, had apparently sent Erica along to me.

The commonest reason for someone being eaten alive in their own home is the death of a cat. Fleas live in carpets, hopping on to the resident pet when in need of food. As long as Tiddles remains hale and hearty, humans are bitten only sporadically. But a few weeks after a feline departure, the now-starving fleas start to feast on the grieving owner, leaping on to their legs as they walk past. Erica, however, denied any previous pet ownership. And flea bites are typically clustered around the ankles and lower shins, whereas Erica said she was affected all over.

'May I?' I asked, taking her hand. I scrutinised the skin of her wrist, and the web spaces between her fingers. Infestation with scabies is surprisingly common, and those are favourite locations for the mites. There was nothing to see, though, and nor did any of the red lumps on her forearms display the hairline tracks that scabies mites make when burrowing through the skin.

It wasn't just Erica's hands that were spared involvement. While most of her torso was scratched and bump-strewn, her mid-back was blemish-free. This pattern suggests something called prurigo. Incessant scratching of normal skin results in the development of raised red prurigo lumps, which can easily be mistaken for insect bites. The area between the shoulder-blades remains unaffected, though, because it is impossible concertedly to scratch there.

'I think we'd better check some blood tests,' I told Erica. There's a host of medical conditions that can cause generalised itch, from iron-deficiency through to underactive thyroid. I gave her prescription for a large bottle of Eurax to be going on with – a fantastic lotion which will suppress itch whatever the cause.

A week later and all the tests were back and normal. Erica was back, too. And this time she'd brought specimens of the offending insects to show me.

'There!' she announced, handing me a little glass jar. I held it up to the light. Inside were a couple of wisps of dark fluff, and some indeterminate bits of debris such as might be found on anyone's floor. Not even tapping the contents on to my palm for a sift-through could produce any evidence of life forms.

Something about the little glass jar rang a bell. The 'match-box sign' describes the tendency of a particular sort of patient to bring spurious evidence in a small container to show the doctor. I looked at Erica afresh. In her late 50s, a trifle eccentric but absolutely no history or indication of any mental or physical illness. I wondered if she might represent a case of Ekbom's syndrome, or delusional parasitosis.

Delusional parasitosis is a fixed but false belief that one is infested with some sort of parasite, usually an insect. In all other respects, the patient is functioning entirely normally, so presents a convincing account of their troubles to pest control personnel, doctors and veterinarians. As in Erica's case, only when all usual avenues have been exhausted does the truth begin to emerge. A big problem with Ekbom's is the characteristic refusal of the sufferer to accept that they are suffering from a mental illness – they're absolutely convinced they're infested. Antipsychotic drugs, usually employed in schizophrenia, can be very effective, but most Ekbom's patients reject them out of hand, and indeed can become quite irate at the suggestion that there's anything wrong with their mind.

'I'd like you to try these tablets,' I told Erica. 'If you read the leaflet you'll find they're usually used to treat schizophrenia, but bizarrely enough they're also quite likely to reduce the itch and the rash you're experiencing.' I smiled, hoping she wouldn't probe my explanation. I wasn't lying as such; just being very careful which bits of the picture I painted.

She returned a month later and, to my relief, had taken the tablets. 'It's amazing,' she told me, 'it's completely better.' She showed me a few areas of pristine skin and we exchanged words of relief that her ordeal was at an end. Then she fell silent for a few moments. When she spoke again her voice was lowered, embarrassed. 'Doctor, was I psychotic?'

'Well, yes,' I told her, and explained about Ekbom's syndrome. With recovery had come full insight, and she recounted, with something akin to awe, how she now looked at the specimens she'd collected and could see they were nothing but fluff, but could clearly remember perceiving them as dead insects at the time. And the persistent sensation of things crawling over her skin had been utterly real to her.

Ekbom's is fascinating and relatively rare – I doubt I'll see another case. It strikes me that pest control officers, given the nature of their job, must encounter it more often. I imagine they have a cut-off – perhaps two failed fumigations, or when the homeowner starts to present them with bits of debris in a matchbox – when they suggest that a doctor might be better placed to help with this particular infestation.

NEEDLES AND HAY

ACCORDING TO ONE adage, general practice is like looking for a needle in a haystack. The needle is 'proper pathology' - the stuff you'll find in medical textbooks. The haystack is the bewildering array of nebulous complaints that people bring to their doctors: aches, fatigue, palpitations, nausea, rashes, dizziness, numbness ... the list goes on. These symptoms could all signify something serious, yet much of the time they don't amount to anything that could be given a diagnostic label.

I don't agree with the adage, though. It implies that a GP's *raison d'être* is to find needles, whereas helping people make sense of their particular haystack is just as important. Nevertheless, every now and then we will come across a sharp-pointed steel sliver. We need to be continuously alert to spot it before it pricks our metaphorical fingers.

Tim was one of my registrars - a younger doctor I was training. Cheryl was a patient he'd seen on several occasions. She had just turned forty, yet she had markedly raised blood pressure and, try as he might, Tim couldn't get it under control. I joined him for the next consultation - he wanted advice about what to add to the cocktail of medications Cheryl was already taking - and the longer it went on the more intrigued I became.

It was mid-October and, even though we'd had a fine English summer, most people were once again pale. Not so

Cheryl. Of course, sun is never more than an EasyJet flight away, but on closer inspection there was an unusual grey tinge to Cheryl's tan. I scrutinised her more carefully. Her forearms, visible below rolled-up sleeves, were hirsute. Conversely, her head hair was subtly thinning in a 'male pattern' – at crown and at temples. And even though it fitted with her cheerful manner, her facial complexion was distinctly ruddy. As Tim closed the consultation I asked Cheryl if she would mind undertaking some tests.

The pituitary gland is a pea-sized organ buried deep within the brain. It releases a variety of hormones that orchestrate our growth, metabolism, and reproduction. When a benign tumour (adenoma) arises, its cells pump out far too much of their particular hormone. One, ACTH (adrenocorticotropic hormone), stimulates the production of steroids in the adrenal glands. An ACTH-secreting adenoma sends the adrenals into overdrive, the excess steroids eventually wrecking havoc – thinning bones, provoking cataracts, elevating blood pressure, precipitating diabetes, and causing heart disease – something called Cushing's Disease.

Cushing's Disease affects just ten in every million people in the UK each year, so the majority of doctors will never encounter a case in their entire working lives. The secondary conditions it presents with – high blood pressure, diabetes, and so on – are, on the other hand, as common as muck. Rarely do they have an underlying cause. All this means that Cushing's is extremely difficult to diagnose. What had rung a bell for me was a fascinating fact I'd learned decades before at medical school. As well as driving the adrenals, ACTH has the side-effect of stimulating pigment cells in the skin. People with Cushing's Disease have unaccountable tans.

I explained my suspicions to Tim after Cheryl had left. He wasn't convinced. Cheryl's unusual tan could easily have been induced by a sun bed, or come from a bottle. And he hadn't spotted the hair and facial signs that were also suggestive. Laboratory confirmation takes weeks. Finally, the biochemistry consultant rang to say, yes, Cushing's it was. Most doctors get a thrill when they pull off a rare diagnosis. And most other doctors are slightly envious of a colleague who performs such a feat – the consultant wanted to hear the whole story of how I'd come to suspect it.

As for the doctor who has been sifting through the hay and who failed to spot the needle, it can be painful. Things look so neat and so obvious when viewed through the retrospectoscope. *Of course* it was Cushing's: that explains why her blood pressure was so difficult to treat. It was a textbook case.

An experience like that could have undermined Tim's confidence. As well as imparting factual knowledge, one of my roles as a trainer is to prepare my registrars to cope with the ups and downs of medical life. To that end, I told Tim the story of a GP who'd been consulted by a male patient with marriage-threatening snoring – another haystack symptom. For over a year the GP had tried in vain to help; even the Ear Nose & Throat specialists had eventually drawn a blank. In desperation, the patient was referred to a sleep clinic. There, a fresh pair of eyes took one look and diagnosed acromegaly, another vanishingly rare condition caused by a pituitary adenoma – this one secreting growth hormone, which enlarges the extremities, including the tongue and jaw, resulting in intractable snoring. The GP who'd failed to spot the (retrospectively) blindingly obvious diagnosis was me.

Both acromegaly and Cushing's Disease can be arrested

by surgery to remove the adenoma. For doctors involved in their diagnosis there are lessons to be learned. When we pick one out we should feel pleased but not proud. When we miss one we should evaluate our performance honestly, but we should not unduly run ourselves down. Occasional needles will always be fiendishly difficult to detect when buried amidst a shed-load of hay.

SECTION

A CCORDING TO MEDICAL folklore, most mental
health crises occur on Friday afternoons. I'm not
sure that's actually the case, but I couldn't help noticing it
was exactly one minute past twelve on the day before the
weekend when the call from the approved social worker was
put through.

'It's about your patient, Maggie Halliwell,' he explained.
'I'm convening a section assessment. What time might you
be available?'

Committal under a section of the Mental Health Act
(MHA) is one of the most weighty responsibilities a doctor
can have: admitting someone, against their will, to a psychiatric hospital, where they will be detained – potentially for
months – while their condition is evaluated and/or treated.
The deprivation of liberty, and the power to enforce treatment, is subject to numerous safeguards, beginning with the
obligation that two independent doctors – one an experienced
psychiatrist; the other, whenever possible, the patient's own
GP – recommend committal.

MHA assessments are also notorious for taking a heck of
a long time to complete. I sat looking at my schedule for the
afternoon: admin for hospital correspondence, phone calls,
prescriptions, and laboratory results; then tutorial with my
registrar followed by full evening surgery. Nowhere were there
two minutes, let alone two whole hours, just lolling around

waiting for some work to come and fill them. Nevertheless, having known Maggie for many years, I would have a valuable perspective, so something would have to give.

The team assembled on the pavement round the corner from Maggie's house, and her community psychiatric nurse (CPN) briefed us on recent events. Maggie's schizophrenia is usually well controlled on anti-psychotic medication, but periodically she decides she no longer needs to take it, with predictable results. We were in one such phase. Neighbours had reported bizarre and inappropriate behaviour earlier in the week. The CPN had responded by coming daily to supervise Maggie taking her tablets. But yesterday she hadn't been able to get in.

Fortunately, Maggie's sister had come down from Birmingham, so access to the house wasn't a problem today. Maggie elected to see us in her bedroom. MHA assessments are always awkward: there's no way a small herd of healthcare professionals can descend on someone's home in such circumstances and not be intimidating. Maggie remained recumbent throughout, defensively chain-smoking, while the five of us stood in an uncomfortable arc around her bed.

To section someone under the MHA, you have to believe they're suffering from a treatable psychiatric condition that endangers their health and safety, and/or the safety of others. You also have to consider whether community treatment or a voluntary admission might be viable alternatives. Key features are insight and capacity: when people are severely unwell they often can't see it; and they don't have the ability to consent to, and cooperate with, the help that's on offer.

Maggie was certainly behaving erratically and expressing odd views, but it quickly became clear to me that she was far from sectionable. Over the years, I've seen her considerably worse, and I've become thoroughly familiar with her idiosyncratic beliefs (the most endearing is her delusion that she suffers from anorexia nervosa, because she'd once read that when anorexics look in the mirror they perceive themselves to be grossly overweight. This is what Maggie experiences, too, whenever she observes her reflection. She remains stubbornly resistant to any suggestion that a BMI of 35, which puts her comfortably in the 'obese' category, in any way undermines the diagnosis).

After a lengthy interview, we adjourned downstairs to arrive at a collective view. Maggie has been sectioned several times in the past, most recently a couple of summers ago when police were called to find her sitting partially clothed in her front garden with a plastic bag over her head. While some of the team were minded to admit her, on the basis of what might happen if she continued to deteriorate, I resisted; these are not sufficient grounds under the MHA. Maggie stayed at home, and gradually stabilised again. The assessment might have trashed my timetable, but it was an afternoon well spent.

CONDOM QUEST

I WAS IN the middle of a tutorial with my registrar when a knock came at the door. One of the other GPs, Liz, poked her head inside.

'Sorry to interrupt,' she said, 'but have you got any condoms?'

I looked at her. Her hair was in its usual neat pony tail, and nothing about her complexion hinted at passions aroused. Nevertheless, an opportunity had clearly arisen that she'd decided she couldn't allow to pass. I pride myself on being open-minded. I only hoped it was with a fellow staff member rather than a patient.

'Oh! No!' she laughed, it suddenly dawning on her how her request had sounded. 'I'm trying to do a coil. The vaginal walls keep prolapsing.'

Coils are a popular 'fit and forget' method of contraception. They're introduced through the cervix and sit in the cavity of the womb, preventing pregnancy for five years. In order to insert one, the doctor passes a duck-billed instrument called a speculum. When the speculum blades are fully opened, the cervix can be accessed at the top of the vagina – except in occasional cases like the one Liz was contending with, where the vaginal walls were extremely lax and kept folding in to the space created by the opening blades, obscuring her view.

These days, with virtually all surgeries staffed by GPs of both sexes, family planning is invariably dealt with by female doctors, so I'd never encountered this problem. Nor had I come across the trick to get round it. Liz explained that you cut the end off a condom, creating a 'sleeve' to slide over the speculum, which then holds back the prolapsing walls to allow proper access.

'We might just have some,' I told her, and we set off for the treatment room. A decade ago, the practice participated in something called the C-Card Scheme. Young people were issued with 'condom cards' at schools and youth clubs, with which they could obtain free prophylactics. The idea was to reduce teenage pregnancy and sexual infection by removing the cost of buying condoms. Like many well-meaning schemes, however, C-Cards failed to take off. To a teenager, making a nurse appointment for such purposes simply screamed I'M GOING TO HAVE SEX! and was therefore ground-swallowingly embarrassing. There was a chance we still had the unused stocks somewhere.

None of the nurses were around, so Liz and I started to search the treatment room cupboards. These are like a museum of failed public health initiatives. There were some old 'portion plates' - plastic crockery divided into segments labelled for meat (small), potatoes/pasta (small), and vegetables (large). We found bundles of leaflets left over from drives to encourage exercise, and inform about safe drinking. Just as I was about to give up, I glimpsed a box right at the back of the top shelf. A life-size rubber model of an erect phallus was poking out. I felt a moment of sympathy for my nursing colleagues: this is what they'd been supposed to use to educate the youth of the district in the proper application of a condom.

Although the nurses had kept hold of the model penis, the box proved to be otherwise empty.

'Would a glove do?' I asked Liz.

'Maybe,' she said. 'But they aren't usually stretchy enough.'

I thought the gloves that came inside our wound dressing packs were thinner and more pliable than the standard examination ones, so we went down the corridor. We were just entering the storeroom when one of our nurses came along.

'Oh, Andrea,' I said. 'Do you know if we still have any condoms?'

Her expression must have mirrored mine earlier. The sight of Liz and me heading into a darkened storeroom, begging passers-by for contraceptives.

Liz told me later that the glove hadn't worked, so she'd had to refer her patient to the family planning clinic. But the 'condom quest' lives on in our surgery's folklore today.

NEAD

DAYTIME EMERGENCIES ARE always disruptive – patients with appointments end up waiting for ages, and hard-pressed colleagues have to squeeze extras into already congested lists to deal with the backlog. So when 70-year-old Brendan's son was put through in the middle of morning surgery, I took the call with some foreboding.

'Dad's having another fit,' he told me. 'I was going to phone the ambulance, but the hospital told us to ring you if it happened again.'

At that stage, I didn't know Brendan or his situation, but this struck me as unusual advice, so I speed-read the last hospital letter on his notes. He'd had three 'blue light' admissions with fits, but the consensus was that they weren't epilepsy. The provisional diagnosis was pseudoseizures, and it was suggested that emergency admission would not be appropriate for future episodes. Brendan's son sounded understandably stressed. I was going to have to visit.

Brendan was still fitting when I arrived, a bizarre pattern of involuntary writhing and inarticulate speech quite different to classical epilepsy. I was able to get him to cooperate with some instructions in the midst of it all, a finding also inconsistent with an ordinary seizure. I put the restive waiting room out of my mind, and settled down to resolve the crisis by persistent reassurance.

Pseudoseizures – less pejoratively known as non-epileptic

attack disorder, or NEAD – are a type of conversion illness: strange phenomena in which intolerable emotional stresses are manifest as dramatic physical symptoms that don't fit organic patterns. These include paralysis and mutism as will be familiar to readers of Pat Barker's *Regeneration* trilogy, which dealt with 'shell shock' in First World War combatants.

In the months that followed, I got to know Brendon well. He'd never served in the military, but his work with an international NGO had landed him in some sticky situations, including being held hostage at gunpoint during an African civil war in the seventies. His personal life had been marred by tragedy: he'd fathered his son during an affair with a married woman, whom he described as the love of his life. She'd died from cancer two years afterwards and her scandalised family had barred him from visiting her during her final months, so he never got to say goodbye.

Brendan is well-educated and professed himself fascinated by my idea that his fits might be related to these past traumas. He is also pretty much the archetype of the stiff-upper-lipped Briton, and courteous with it, so he was very polite in telling me he thought the whole thing was a load of hogwash. He undertook vast amounts of research, which reinforced his belief that he must have an unusual variant of epilepsy. His conviction wasn't shaken by either a second opinion from a nationally renowned neurological centre, or a fruitless trial of epilepsy medication.

Brendan's fits escalated, coming several times a day, disrupting life to such an extent that he could barely leave the house. He started to fear that he wouldn't be able to attend his son's wedding planned for the following year. With great reluctance, he finally agreed to pursue psychological therapy, the only modality to have any efficacy in NEAD.

The initial course was at a regional specialist centre in a nearby city. Their approach was heavily behavioural, which Brendan experienced as deeply patronising, and I was dismayed as relations between him and his therapists irretrievably broke down. I started to fear that he would be among the two-thirds of NEAD patients unable to benefit from treatment. Over the months, though, a bond of trust had developed between us, which must have played a part in his accepting my suggestion of a further referral to a national expert in NEAD psychological therapy at a psychiatric hospital in a distant city – the funding for which I had to go to considerable lengths to secure.

Brendan's son ferried him to and from the appointments over a sixteen-week period, and to all our delight, his fits – which had been going on for eighteen months by then – gradually petered out. He eventually managed to witness his son, whose mother he had loved so much, get married. For all the disruption, I'm glad I went on that urgent home visit, which started Brendan and me on the long road to his eventual cure.

OUT OF HOURS

VERONICE

I FIRST CAME across Veronice a couple of years ago, when I was on duty at the out-of-hours service.

'I'm a diabetic,' she told me, 'and I'm feeling really poorly.' She detailed a litany of symptoms. I said I'd be round straightaway.

What sounded worrying on the phone proved very different in her smoke-fugged sitting room. She was comfortable, chatty, had no fever or sign of illness, and her blood sugar was well controlled. In fact, she looked remarkably well. As I tried to draw the visit to a close, she began to regale me with complaints about her own GP: how he neglected her needs, dismissed her symptoms, refused to take her calls.

It sounded unlikely, but I listened sympathetically and with an open mind. Bit by bit, other professionals were brought into the frame: persecutory social workers, vindictive housing officers, corrupt policemen, and a particularly odious psychiatrist who'd had her locked up in hospital for months, and had recently discharged her to live in this new, hateful bungalow. By the time she'd told me about her sit-in at the local newspaper's offices – to try to force them to cover her story – and described her attempts to be arrested so she could go to court and tell a judge about the whole saga, it was clear Veronice wasn't interacting with the world in quite the same way as the rest of us.

It's a delicate path to tread, extricating oneself from such a situation. The mental health issues could safely be left to her usual daytime team to follow up, so my task was to get out of the door without further inflaming the perceptions of neglect and maltreatment. It didn't go too well to start with. Her voice got louder and louder: was I, too, going to do nothing to help? Couldn't I see she was really ill? I'd be sorry when she didn't wake up the next morning.

What worked fantastically was asking her what she actually wanted me to do. Her first stab – to get her re-housed back to her old area as an emergency that evening – was so beyond the plausible that even she seemed able to accept my protestations of impotence. When I asked her again, all the heat suddenly went out of her voice. She said she didn't think she had any food; could I get her something to eat? A swift check revealed a fridge and cupboards stocked with the basics. I gave her some menu suggestions, but drew the line at preparing the meal myself. By then, she seemed meekly willing to allow me to go.

We've had many out-of-hours conversations since. For all her strangeness, she is wily, and knows the medical gambits to play in order to trigger a home visit. Having been conned into another couple of fruitless house calls, I now parry the proffered symptoms and generally get to the heart of the matter on the phone. It usually revolves around food. Could I bring some bread and milk? She's got no phone credit left; could I ring the Chinese and order her a home delivery?

She came up on the screen again recently. I rang, to be told about excruciating ear pain, discharge, and fever. I sighed, accepting defeat: with that story I had no choice but to go round. I popped to the drug cupboard first, though.

Predictably enough, I found normal temperature, pristine ears, glucose fine, Veronice smiling away.

'Well,' I said, 'whatever's causing your ear to hurt is a medical mystery. Take some paracetamol and it'll be fine in the morning.'

There was a flash of triumph in her eyes. 'Ah, but doctor, I haven't got any. Could you—'

Before she could finish, I produced a pack of paracetamol from my jacket pocket. I detected a look of first surprise, then real admiration, as I dropped it in her lap. She may have succeeded in suckering me round again, but I'd second-guessed her. I was out of the door in under five minutes. A score draw.

POSTER GIRL

ANTHONY, MY REGISTRAR, took an out-of-hours call from a care home. One of the residents, a twenty-five-year-old named Daryl, was complaining of pain in his nether-regions. The nurse said his testicles looked very swollen. It sounded like a straightforward infection, and Anthony was happy to go on his own. However, as part of the box-ticking necessary to complete his training, he needed his proficiency in male genital examination to be witnessed and signed-off. This would be a perfect opportunity, so I came along too.

The care home is tucked away in a nearby village – I don't have any patients there myself, but I've sometimes visited out-of-hours. The front is an Edwardian house, but there's a sprawling 1950s block on the back, with wide, echoey, linoleum-floored corridors leading to several dozen residents' rooms. These are people with complex disabilities that render independent living impracticable: paralysis following spinal trauma, severe multiple sclerosis, motor neurone disease. They have precious little autonomy left, and the care staff have made great efforts to cheer up the austere institutional surroundings – each bedroom is chock-full of personal effects and mementoes.

Daryl had been paralysed below the waist in a motorcycle accident. He'd also sustained a brain injury that left him with a mental ability akin to a five-year-old. I watched patiently as

Anthony tried to gain his consent to be examined. Just like a young child, Daryl was scared of doctors. He kept interrupting Anthony, shaking his hand and asking him repetitious questions – where did he live? what was his favourite colour? – in heartbreakingly transparent attempts to divert the conversation on to safer ground. Eventually, with the help of Linda, a familiar and trusted nurse, Anthony managed to gain Daryl's confidence, and set about confirming the diagnosis.

It wasn't an infection. The apparent testicular swelling was because of a huge mass in his perineum (the area behind the scrotum) which was displacing everything forwards. Neither Anthony nor I had encountered such a thing before. The likeliest explanation was an abscess, but its texture felt ominously tumour-like. Either way, Daryl needed to be admitted to hospital.

Gaining Daryl's consent to examination was one thing, getting his agreement to go to hospital quite another. Despite Linda and Anthony's best efforts, he became increasingly stressed – shaking hands, wanting kisses, asking again and again about favourite colours. Just then, I noticed a poster on the wall facing Daryl's bed. It was a blow-up of a photo of him with two young women. I was intrigued to recognise the one on his left: a patient of mine, a lovely, gentle lass called Megan. I asked Daryl about the picture. Megan is his sister, he told me. Amazing, I said, I know her really well; she often brings her kids in to see me. We talked more about her: what a kind person she is, how funny she can be, how much Daryl loves her.

Within a short time, Daryl had visibly relaxed. I told him that, if Megan were here, she would want him to go to hospital to get help. He thought about this for a while, then – much to our relief – nodded, and agreed she would. He held my hand and kissed it. I'd seen enough of his way of connecting with people to be sure of my ground, so I gave his hand a kiss in return.

Fortunately, the tumour, while rare, turned out to be benign. After a short spell in hospital, Daryl returned to the home. How much more distressing the admission would have been for him, had it not been for the poster on his wall, and the chance presence of a doctor who happened to recognise his beloved sibling.

SAFEGUARDING

THE CALL CAME on Sunday evening, flagged as urgent on the computer. I rang the home number, which was answered by a woman.

'My father is dying of prostate cancer with bony mets,' she explained. 'He's in a lot of pain.'

The medical terminology struck me. 'Are you in healthcare?'

'I'm a nurse. I don't mean to tell you your job, but I think it's time for a syringe driver.'

As death approaches, medication taken by mouth can become unreliable. In order to control symptoms, drugs are administered subcutaneously by a device known as a syringe driver. The siting of a driver often heralds the final hours of life. As well as relieving pain and mental distress, the potent drugs used can depress consciousness and respiration, which more often than not hastens the end. This is not euthanasia: it is permissible as the price of effective palliation, the 'doctrine of double-effect'.

When I arrived at the house, Frank was alone with his daughter, Jill, a neatly dressed woman in her forties who'd travelled down from her Northumberland home to nurse him in his final illness. She described how, no matter how much morphine she gave, she didn't seem able to control his pain. Frank was indeed in a bad way: semi-conscious, markedly confused and rambling, but he didn't appear objectively to be suffering. There was one moment when he did briefly wince.

Jill responded instantaneously, spooning in a dose of liquid morphine as a parent might feed a baby.

'How much has he been having?'

Jill shrugged. 'I give him some every time he's in pain.'

When working out-of-hours one has no access to patients' records – all information has to be gained first-hand. I asked to see the rest of Frank's medication. In the depths of a laden carrier bag I found plenty of paracetamol and diclofenac, an anti-inflammatory.

'What's he having of these?' I asked.

'Oh, nothing,' she told me, 'he's just on oramorph now.'

Bone pain doesn't generally respond to morphine alone. One usually prescribes paracetamol and anti-inflammatories; they potentiate the effect of morphine, allowing far less opiate to be used. I wrote out a schedule, specifying regular doses of the two abandoned drugs, and insisting that Jill note down every dose of oramorph given.

It had all taken a long time. Leaving, I bumped into two other women coming in the gate, who turned out to be Frank's elderly wife with another daughter. I'd had no idea there was a spouse around. She seemed equally bewildered to meet me, saying her daughter had taken her out for an evening drive. It was mid-winter and dark outside.

The overdosing on morphine was one thing; quite another was the removal of Frank's wife before calling the doctor in. Safeguarding children is a familiar concept, but in recent years there's been a growing realisation that adults are sometimes comparably vulnerable and in need of protection. I contacted Frank's GP first thing in the morning, and he convened an urgent safeguarding conference. A troubling picture emerged. Frank's four children had a lifelong history of rivalry, division, and competition for paternal attention. Jill and her sister were allies against the other two, and against their mother. The wider family reported that Jill had descended on the home, taking control of Frank's treatment and shutting the others out, pulling rank by virtue of her spell in nursing some fifteen years before.

The conference prohibited Jill from further direct involvement in Frank's care. Treatment optimised, Frank came off virtually all morphine. His confusion resolved completely, and he had another five months of good quality life. Whatever her motivations – and whether she had even been consciously aware of them – Jill had been hastening his demise. How easy it would have been for an out-of-hours doctor unwittingly to have colluded – taking things at face-value in the absence of knowledge of the situation and the family dynamics, and acceding to Jill's suggestion that the time for a syringe driver was nigh.

ANAPHYLAXIS

THE OUT-OF-HOURS RECEPTIONIST, Gaby, came and found me while I was still setting up for the evening shift. A patient had arrived unexpectedly early for their appointment, she told me, but rather than him waiting to be seen, Gaby thought she ought to let me know he was 'swelling up, and finding it hard to breathe.'

I glanced at the summary from the III call handler: the problem was supposed to have been a sore throat. Nothing about swelling or breathlessness at all. I hurried along to the waiting room.

Jay turned out to be in his early twenties, accompanied by a concerned neighbour and a massive bag full of medication. He wasn't able to explain much about what was happening; he seemed preoccupied with taking each laboured breath. His lips were huge and rubbery. He indicated a rubber Medic-Alert bracelet round his wrist. 'Chronic angioedema,' it read, along with a list of half a dozen medications that mustn't be administered.

During the few moments it took to gather these first impressions, Jay's inspirations developed a disconcerting 'whoop', and his breathing rate plummeted. He sagged sideways in his chair. It never fails to feel slightly surreal when you suddenly realise you're in a life-and-death situation – Jay was steaming full-speed towards a respiratory arrest. Through the clear plastic of his carrier bag, I spotted the bright orange boxes of no less than four Epipens – syringes pre-filled with doses of adrenaline.

'Has he had any?' I asked his neighbour.

He looked as alarmed as I felt. 'No.'

I shelled one of the Epipens out. They're brilliant bits of kit: you flip a protective cover off the top, press with your thumb, then stab the other end hard against the patient's thigh. That fires a needle through clothing, skin and into muscle, whereupon the device injects life-saving hormone. It functioned like a dream. With the neighbour's help, I then got Jay horizontal and shoved his legs in the air, to boost the blood pressure that – had I had the time to measure it – would have been somewhere in the region of his boots.

Gaby was dispatched to phone 999 for an ambulance, and I stayed monitoring while the adrenaline did its miraculous work. Within a couple of minutes, Jay's breathing had eased, his lip swelling was subsiding, and he was able to speak to assure me he was much improved. I filled in some of the story. This was the umpteenth time he'd developed anaphylaxis – an acute onset, rapidly fatal, whole-body allergic reaction. Most often it's caused by insect stings or food allergies, but Jay has an extremely rare variant whereby simple, common infections trigger the same calamitous response. His drug bag contained all manner of steroids, antihistamines, and other allergy-suppressant tablets, which he took on a daily basis to try to prevent it happening. They didn't seem to be doing a very good job.

The thing that mystified me was why he hadn't self-administered an Epipen and called 999 when he'd realised what was happening. It seemed a great example of cognitive dissonance. At one level, he knew he should have done, but he so hated having to be repeatedly admitted to hospital that he'd somehow convinced himself that he'd be able to head off the impending crisis with an increased dose of steroids.

The only place for someone with anaphylaxis is hospital – while adrenaline is life-saving, it can wear off quite quickly. Patients need to be monitored until it's certain that the allergic reaction has been fully suppressed. Anyone who doubts that the NHS is overstretched should try phoning for an ambulance round here. Twenty-five minutes elapsed with no sign of flashing blue lights. Jay's lips started ballooning again, and his breathing began to deteriorate. Another Epipen. Another call to ambulance control. Another twenty-five minutes before a crew – who had had to come from about 50 miles away – arrived.

Jay safely dispatched to hospital, I congratulated Gaby on her quick thinking in coming to fetch me. I myself was more than a little adrenaline-pumped, something Gaby kindly treated with a large infusion of tea.

THE LAST GAMBLE

M Y NEW REGISTRAR, Caroline, rang the bell, and we waited together in the winter evening's drizzle. A few moments later, the door was opened by a neatly dressed woman in her late sixties, her face etched with anxiety.

'Thank goodness you're here!'

'You sounded very worried about your mother on the phone,' Caroline said as we stepped inside.

'Yes, frightened, in fact.'

Caroline and I exchanged a look as we walked along the hall. People describing themselves as frightened are communicating a whole different level of concern. This lady's elderly mother was likely to be very sick indeed.

I was surprised, then, to find a spry-looking woman sitting in the fireside chair. She gave us a grin, and waved a cheery hand in greeting. Her breathing rate was elevated, admittedly, but initial impressions were starkly at odds with her daughter's degree of anxiety.

I observed while Caroline took a history. It turned out that their own doctor had visited during the day and diagnosed a chest infection. The antibiotics he'd prescribed were an appropriate choice, but they wouldn't have started to work yet. I listened while Caroline tried to uncover the reason for the out-of-hours visit request, but there seemed to have been no deterioration or new symptoms to have prompted the urgent call-out.

While Caroline conducted her examination, the daughter remained hovering in the doorway, her hands clasped tight with worry. The mother was running a fever as expected, but her oxygen saturations were good, likewise her blood pressure. There was no mental confusion. Everything looked essentially satisfactory. I was increasingly puzzled as to why we'd been called round.

I glanced at the notes print-out. Mother and daughter had the same surname, meaning the daughter was probably unmarried. They lived together, and I wondered if the daughter had never left home. That would suggest a very close relationship. Perhaps that explained her degree of fear – the prospect of losing the maternal figure she'd lived with her whole life.

I noted the mother's year of birth: ninety-nine years old. Aiming to ease the tension, I made a light-hearted remark about getting a card from the Queen next birthday. It provoked a whole spiel from the daughter: how you'd have thought there would have been an automatic process for Buckingham Palace to identify upcoming centenarians, but when the daughter had been in touch with them she'd found there wasn't, so she'd had to make them aware of her mother's impending anniversary herself. My puzzlement deepened. The birthday was still nine months away. The daughter was coming across as ever-more neurotic, badgering officialdom so far in advance of her mum's landmark celebration. I couldn't work out what was going on.

'I expect you're planning quite a party,' I said, while Caroline was stowing her equipment in her bag.

'I should say,' the daughter agreed. She mentioned the country house hotel they'd booked – one of the area's poshest. They'd already had a dry-run, she told us, inviting guests to the house to check her mother would have the stamina for it.

Caroline reassured them that the infection should soon resolve with the treatment already commenced, and expressed the hope that they enjoy the party when the day came. Mother and daughter exchanged a conspiratorial smile and, after a pause, confessed that William Hill was going to be paying for the lavish do.

We listened with increasing amusement as they explained that, twenty years previously, they'd put £100 on the mother living to receive her centenary greeting from the Queen. The odds quoted at the time had been very long. As year after year of good health had passed, the payout – set to be over ten thousand pounds – had gone from whimsical fantasy to tangible reality. All mum had to do was hang on another nine months.

Caroline and I had a wry debrief on the way back to base. The prospect of losing a loved parent was bad enough, but the daughter evidently found any illness now to be intolerably worrying, threatening as it did to rob them of their audacious winnings just as the final hurdle hoved into sight.

CHICKEN UNGA FEVER

E VERY FEW YEARS in our new-look, semi-privatised NHS, the contract for running our out of hours service changes from one commercial provider to another. One such takeover – by a firm I'll call the Big Beast of the North – resulted in policies and procedures being dictated by faceless managers located several hundred miles away. One of their first actions was severely to restrict doctors' access to the internet from the desktop PCs in the out-of-hours centre, presumably because they feared we were spending our time posting on Facebook, or auctioning second-hand diagnostic equipment on eBay, rather than attending to patients.

Computers play an increasingly central role in medical care. Anyone seeking assistance outside normal hours is now filtered through the 111 service, where they will speak to call-centre staff operating a piece of software called NHS Pathways. NHS Pathways prompts these non-clinical call-handlers to ask what is often a protracted series of questions, at the end of which the programme generates a 'disposition' that tells the operator what to do. In the most urgent of scenarios this might be to phone an ambulance, or to tell the patient to attend A&E. Less pressing problems are dealt with by the advice to contact their GP the next day. Intermediate-level issues result in the caller's details being sent electronically to an out-of-hours doctor, together with a summary of the case.

I have great sympathy for the 111 staff. The world of

medicine is replete with strange vocabulary: baffling drug names, weird diagnostic labels, and other arcane terminology. With a bare minimum of training, the non-clinical call handlers are plunged into the fray, and their efforts to make sense of what they're hearing frequently end in endearing misinterpretations of what the patient has told them.

It's usually possible to work things out from the context. 'Sis tightus' means a bladder infection (cystitis), 'Simba Statin' is actually a cholesterol-lowering drug (simvastatin), and the enigmatic 'Angie O'Gram' turns out to be a procedure to investigate heart disease.

One evening, though, I was stumped by a request to ring a patient who had apparently been diagnosed with 'Chicken Unga Fever'. It's impossible for any one person to know everything in medicine, and I wondered if a new variant of bird flu had escaped my notice. It's never good to contact a patient from a position of ignorance, so I set about trying to gen up before making the call.

Having been blocked from accessing all but a very limited set of approved medical websites, I tried putting 'Chicken Unga Fever' into the search box of each of them but returned precisely no matches. Fortunately, our new managers in the north-east had yet to figure out how to stop doctors carrying smartphones, so I called up Google on mine, and set it to the task. Within a fraction of a second it was asking me if I really meant 'Chikungunya fever'? It was not a condition I'd encountered before, but it sounded promising, so I did some rapid reading. It turned out to be a nasty viral infection that is transmitted, like malaria, by mosquitos. As such it is endemic in Africa and Asia and, with global warming, it is now prevalent in the Caribbean – where my patient had contracted it – and is spreading into the United States and southern Europe.

The main problem with chikungunya is a crippling arthritis, the virus directly attacking the cartilage that lines joints. Symptoms can persist for months or even years after the initial infection. This was indeed what my patient was experiencing, and I was now in a position to advise medication to control the pain and inflammation. Chikungunya can also present with mild haemorrhagic symptoms, a bit like a minor version of Ebola, so it was also reassuring to learn that the virus cannot spread without the mosquito vector, meaning there was no risk to anyone here in the UK, and in any case rarely proves fatal.

The experience reinforced for me the centrality of the web in medical life. Upstairs in my surgery, we are gradually disposing of the many hundreds of textbooks in the practice library, the vast majority of which we now never refer to. Online learning, and the power of Google, are here to stay. Health service managers need a more creative response than imposing arbitrary internet restrictions on clinicians practising in the modern world.

IN HOURS

HECTOR

WHEN VISITING PATIENTS at home, I generally ask for any dogs to be shut in another part of the house. Unlike cats, who usually ignore strangers, the arrival of an unfamiliar man is of supreme interest to any canine. The more protective and territorial breeds leap straight to DefCon 1. Many's the consultation I've had to conduct above the barking and snarling of an incensed hound, bashing itself against a perilously thin panelled door in a determined effort to get its teeth into the intruder.

Smaller breeds tend to be more friendly - though most Labradors are also fairly genial - but this poses its own problems. Dogs are intensely olfactory animals, and a new human brings an enticing smorgasbord of aromas to investigate. It is difficult to maintain a professional interest in a patient's breathing difficulties while having repeatedly to remove Fido's snout from one's crotch.

One exception to my no-dogs rule was Hector, a white miniature poodle belonging to Gordon and Irene Ives. Gordon spent several years housebound with end-stage heart failure, and he was regularly on the list for a home visit. Hector became accustomed to doctors and district nurses calling, and would greet each arrival with a charming display of excited rushing around, tail wagging nineteen to the dozen. Once the initial thrill had subsided, he would settle himself on the sofa next to you, contentedly being stroked while you discussed

Gordon's symptoms and charted his slow but inexorable decline.

There were two occasions when Gordon actually died, Irene's frantic 999 calls bringing paramedics in time successfully to restart his heart. Irene told me Hector seemed to recognise the dramatic difference in these situations, and kept out of the way of the resuscitation efforts.

Gordon spent many months living on borrowed time before the third episode of fatal arrhythmia from which he could not be brought back. We feared for Irene's emotional health. For years her existence had centred around caring for Gordon, and now suddenly he was gone. She had always been somewhat anxious, periodically depending on mild tranquillisers for her 'nerves', and following her bereavement she developed agoraphobia, which made it impossible to attend surgery. My home visits continued, now focused on helping her through this difficult period. Hector remained as ebullient as ever, and there was a difficult disconnect between his playful bouncing on and off the furniture while I tried to support Irene in her grief and dislocation.

Eventually, though, things improved, and I began to see less of Irene. When she did require attention, she would make an appointment. I always enquired after Hector, and her expression, and the way she talked about so fondly about him, bespoke of the comfort he gave. His need for walks had gradually restored her confidence in going out, and he was an irrepressibly sunny companion in the otherwise empty house.

Irene came to see me just after I'd got back from holiday one summer. I was sad to learn that Hector had died while I'd been away. It was something we'd discussed among the team: what would happen to Irene if she lost her dog as well.

Far from a resurgence of grief, however, she told me her overwhelming feeling was of relief. Now in her early 80s, she'd become increasingly worried by the thought of what would happen to Hector were she to pre-decease him. She confessed to having become preoccupied by disturbing visions of him alone in the house, perplexed, nudging and worrying at her lifeless body. As it was, he'd lived out his days in his inimitable style, and had been put peacefully to sleep once the vet had diagnosed cancer.

Irene misses him, of course, but there's been no recurrence of her anxiety or agoraphobia – something we'd thought would likely happen. She seems to have drawn strength from no longer having to worry about his future. At some point, though, I'm bound to do another visit to her home, and it will be strange not to meet Hector there.

MARTHA

MARTHA MADE AN appointment soon after moving to our area, seeking antibiotics for a malodorous vaginal discharge. It was a recurrent problem, she told me, and her previous doctor used to give her courses of metronidazole, which would clear it up just fine, albeit only temporarily.

In her late thirties, she had baggy combats and several piercings. There was a palpable tension about her. I reassured her she could see a female GP if she'd prefer, or could have a chaperone present for any examination. That wouldn't be necessary, she told me, because she couldn't allow anyone – male or female – to examine her. We talked a bit more, and she told me about the sexual abuse she'd experienced as a child. She had managed one sexual relationship many years earlier, but it had lasted just six months before foundering on her extreme phobia of intimate contact.

I had every sympathy with her old GP. Faced with an inability properly to investigate her problem, he and Martha had fallen into a pragmatic conspiracy. Metronidazole brought short-term relief, so that was what she kept being given. I was uneasy, though. I explained that we needed somehow to check her cervix, which necessitates vaginal examination. After a lot of careful negotiation she agreed to an urgent referral.

I briefed the loveliest female gynaecologist in our patch, who handled things with great sensitivity. Ultimately, though, Martha couldn't permit examination, so an urgent MRI scan was arranged instead. The news was not good: there was a huge tumour at the neck of the womb, extending into the pelvis. If this was cervical cancer then it was far beyond the curable stage, but an operation could ameliorate horrendous symptoms from tumour progression. A lymphoma was also a possibility, and this would be more treatable. Either way, Martha was facing a stark choice: to enter a programme of surgery, radiotherapy, and subsequent follow-up checks, every stage of which was going to necessitate doctors examining her in ways she found intolerable; or to suffer an imminent and extremely unpleasant death.

Given months, if not years, a psychologist might have been able to help her overcome her phobia. But there was no time. Terrified, Martha fled to a town some distance away. She remained in phone contact, though, and I did my best to support her as she tried to confront her living nightmare. She developed debilitating panic attacks. The last time we spoke, she mentioned how her breathing had become difficult, a classic physical symptom of morbid anxiety.

The next day she collapsed and died. The post-mortem revealed a blood clot in a leg vein – something more common in cancer patients, especially when a large pelvic mass impedes blood flow. A piece of clot had broken off into her circulation and lodged in her lungs – a pulmonary embolus – with fatal results. I will never know whether her breathing difficulty was really anxiety-related, or if had been due to an earlier, smaller piece of clot. Her tumour was confirmed as advanced cervical cancer; she was never going to have survived. That was the only crumb of comfort in the whole tragedy – that her inevitable death had been swift, and her dignity had been preserved.

Cervical cancer is sexually transmitted, and may well have been caused by a virus contracted from her abuser. It is readily preventable by three-yearly smear tests, but the psychological sequelae of the abuse meant Martha could never contemplate being screened. Sexual abuse in childhood wrecks lives, and in Martha's case it prematurely ended hers.

A friend of hers came to see me after the funeral. She told me that Martha had often mentioned the way I and my gynaecologist colleague had related to her – one of the few times in her life she had felt truly respected. By the time we met Martha it was too late to save her, but the other crumb of comfort is that she found doctors who had done their utmost to treat her with the dignity to which every person should be entitled.

Information about cervical screening services especially for women who have experienced sexual violence can be found at www.mybodybackproject.com

AL FRESCO

O UT-OF-HOURS HAD BEEN busy the night before, and by mid-afternoon I was flagging. Outside, it was one of the first truly summery days of the year. My usual enthusiasm was proving hard to muster; there were just so many patients still to see before I'd be able to get home and rest.

I had mixed feelings when I saw Alan was my next appointment. I'm very fond of him, so I should have been pleased. But what had happened since we last met made me trepidatious about the consultation to come.

Alan and his wife moved here three years ago, after he retired as head of geography at a public school. He was clearly one of those teachers who command pupils' respect. Plain-speaking and sure of his own mind, he exuded confidence, but there was no hint of arrogance or intolerance. He had an unremittingly positive outlook and a great appetite for life. By the time we'd had a few consultations, I knew all about his new house and the rockery he was planning to create in its garden. He loved fly fishing, and he was delighted by the new butterfly species he was encountering while walking the dog. After a while, he joined a community group, and had a mischievous glint in his eye when recounting the latest triumph over bloody-minded bureaucracy. Alan was the sort of man who believed in starting each day with a hearty cooked breakfast.

His health was as robust as his temperament, excepting

the operation he'd had to remove a cancerous kidney. His remaining kidney was functioning fine, but we had to do a fair amount of tinkering with blood pressure medications to get round a tendency to salt imbalance.

Then nine months ago, I received a letter from the hospital saying Alan had presented with frank blood in his urine. A scan had found a new cancer in the second kidney. The only treatment was to remove the diseased organ, condemning him to spend the rest of his life on renal dialysis.

Dialysis entails three long mornings each week up at the hospital, and this, coupled with the complexity of their altered physiology, means that patients tend to be looked after exclusively by the renal physicians. I hadn't seen Alan since. While dialysis keeps people alive, it is common to experience marked fatigue, and symptoms such as muscle cramps and altered appetite, which take their toll on quality of life. The thought of meeting Alan again, and witnessing his inevitable decline – the loss of all those outdoor activities that had given his life meaning – made me sad.

I went to click his name on the screen, and noticed the receptionist's message: 'Sitting on wall outside with dog'. I walked through the waiting room, out of the front door, and found Alan basking in the sunshine with Jess, his black Labrador, at his feet. We quickly decided it was too nice to be cooped up indoors, so I sat myself next to him and we conducted the consultation al fresco.

We dealt with his problem swiftly, then proceeded to catch up. The first months of dialysis had been hard, but he delighted in telling me how well he was now doing. The rockery was finished, he'd resumed dog walks, and was on the brink of returning to the river with his rods. And he did look well.

Today was his seventieth birthday. He'd been for dialysis that morning, and had taken cakes for the staff and other patients, many of whom had become good friends.

As we talked, we provoked broad smiles from patients coming in and out of the surgery. The sun was gloriously warm. I reached down and stroked Jess's head. I could see my receptionist, watching through the glass doors, clearly tickled. By the time Alan and I were done, my enthusiasm and energy had returned in spades. Sometimes our patients give us something unexpected and precious, and there's no better example than Alan.

REFLUX

E LAINE HAD BEEN getting chest pains, and sometimes an unpleasant fluid would arrive at the back of her
throat, scorching the tissues there. It was worse when she lay
down, making getting to sleep difficult.

A few questions ruled out anything sinister, so I gave her
my standard spiel, explaining how our stomachs are able to
withstand their acid contents, but not so our gullets. When
gastric fluid refluxes back up towards the throat it causes a
chemical burn to the lining of the oesophagus. It's a common
problem and easy to treat with proton pump inhibitors (PPIs),
medications that switch off acid production in the stomach.

Even as I rounded off my little speech, though, I was
wondering why it was happening to her. Reflux is frequently
linked to obesity or excess alcohol, but Elaine is pretty much
the perfect weight, and she certainly isn't a boozer. Another
explanation would be a hiatus hernia – where the top of the
stomach gets displaced above the diaphragm – but a first presentation in her mid-fifties seemed unlikely somehow.

There was a moment of silence between us. Before I could
decide how to formulate a further enquiry, Elaine took the
plunge.

'Could it be due to stress?'

I readily agreed – our bodies invariably find some physical
way of expressing emotional turmoil, and reflux oesophagitis
is as good as any. Emboldened, Elaine began to tell her story.

'You remember I told you about my son?'

I must have looked puzzled.

'About how he's using cocaine?'

That rang a bell. She'd mentioned it in passing some months before. Patients do this sometimes – test out a doctor's reaction to something they're troubled or ashamed about, then revisit the problem later if they feel they got a sympathetic reception. I encouraged her to continue.

Elaine described how her son's drug use was out of control. In his mid-twenties, with a promising job in a light engineering firm, he still lived at home. When it first became clear he was taking cocaine, Elaine and her husband issued an ultimatum: stop, or leave home. To start with she thought it had worked. But he continued to come back late, saying he'd been out drinking with mates, yet there was never any alcohol on his breath, and his restlessness and inability to sleep told a different story. It was devastating for her, she told me, to see him ruining himself like this.

In desperation, she had taken control of her son's bank card, trying to choke off his access to drugs. Initially, that tactic, too, had appeared to work. But a month ago he confessed that he'd run up over £700 of debt, and told her that his dealers were now after him for payment. I knew what was coming next, even before she said it. Elaine had already paid off the first £200 for him. And she hadn't told her husband about it all, knowing how strongly he would disagree.

It's one of the most difficult transitions for a parent, finally letting go of one's child and allowing them to learn their own lessons. All the more so if the lessons they seem determined to learn appear self-destructive. But by failing to stick to firm boundaries; by assuming for herself the responsibility of trying to stop him buying drugs; then by baling him out when that didn't work, she was serially denying him the opportunity to grow and mature. Unless she changed tack, she was in danger of producing a young man incapable of taking responsibility for himself.

We talked it though. She already knew, in her heart of hearts, what she had to do. First would be a difficult but vital conversation with her husband. Then the two of them, acting as a united front, would need to decide their boundary and unwaveringly stick to it.

I gave her a prescription for a PPI, but by then it felt almost like an afterthought. The remedy for Elaine's reflux lay not in tablets, but in resolving the mess in which she'd allowed herself to become mired.

RESPITE

MEGAN AND SHAUN'S daughter, Rosie, was born with severe cerebral palsy - her intellect is intact but spasticity affects her muscles, distorting her trunk and contracting her limbs, and rendering her speech slow and barely comprehensible. She is wheelchair-bound and, as she's grown bigger, she's come to need hoisting in and out of bed, chair, bathroom and adapted car. She's intelligent, loves her tech, and is acutely aware of the world beyond her home and her special school. Like most teenagers, Rosie just wants to fit in with peers, and she's really struggled with how profoundly her body prevents her from enjoying the kind of life she would love to be living, and from belonging to a group of firm friends.

A couple of years ago, Rosie began taking out her frustration and anger on her parents - most particularly Megan, Shaun working long hours as an engineer with one of the top motor racing teams. The relationship between mother and daughter became progressively more dysfunctional, Megan feeling bullied and cowed by Rosie's tirades and her aggressive non-cooperation. Practicalities and deep-seated guilt made it hard for Megan to impose effective boundaries on Rosie's behaviour, with the result that Rosie became akin to a tyrant. At an unconscious level, the control she was able to exert over her mother made Rosie feel horribly insecure, so she pushed ever harder, craving a fixed boundary. Megan felt powerless to exert authority, and was filled with self-loathing for the extreme resentment she often harboured towards Rosie.

Things came to a head when Rosie started to refuse school by means of some profoundly challenging behaviour. Care fell 24/7 on Megan's already bowed shoulders. She consulted with me about something trivial, initially presenting the same cheerful coping face that she wears when dealing with the rest of the world. But the façade soon dropped, exposing the miserable entrapment she felt, and the agitated hostility that was overwhelming her. She was desperate to get out, to run away, but was simultaneously paralysed by guilt and obligation, and fear of other people's condemnation were she to leave. Suicide was the only escape she could see, and thoughts of it were increasingly preoccupying her. I wondered about prescribing an antidepressant – the only thing I felt I had to offer as a doctor – but what she badly needed was respite: some time away from Rosie in which to find her self again. Although social services were offering to support this, Shaun was implacably opposed, believing it would be yet another negative experience for Rosie.

We discussed things, and I discovered that as a child Megan had loved holidaying with a maiden aunt in south Wales. I opened the prescribing module on my practice computer and switched to the rarely used free text mode, typing 'A week's break in Pembrokeshire; one to be taken every six to eight weeks.' I printed this out on the standard green NHS FP10 prescription form, signed it, and handed it to Megan with instructions to give it to Shaun and not to take no for an answer.

To my amazement, it worked. Although Shaun continued to dislike the idea, he did grudgingly agree to social services providing care for Rosie to allow Megan a series of respite breaks. Her elderly aunt spoiled her, and for a week at a time she drank deeply of freedom and the chance to be nurtured. She would return from each holiday with her head above water again, and it never quite sank beneath the waves again before the next one came around.

Although the situation still has its difficulties, Rosie eventually returned to school, Megan regained some daily 'me time', and the relationship between them has gradually improved. I saw Megan recently, and she told me that Rosie has just had a change of social worker. In discussing needs with the new incumbent, Megan showed her that FP10 from a couple of years ago. The young social worker expressed surprise that anyone could get holidays prescribed on the NHS, and it tickled Megan no end to explain what it had really been about. She thanked me again for writing it, because her impression was that the new social worker had also taken it very seriously, and had assured her that respite care would continue to be funded. Sometimes the power of a prescription lies not just in the medicine, but in the very words themselves.

WHITE SPOTITIS

I WAS CONSULTED by the Tin Man from the Wizard of Oz recently. He hadn't come about rusted-up joints, though; he had a sore throat.

'When did he become unwell?' I asked his mother.

'Yesterday,' she said. 'I looked in his throat this morning and saw white spots. I think he's got tonsillitis.'

The term tonsillitis literally means 'inflamed tonsils', but both doctors and patients/parents use it to mean something different – a throat infection that needs an antibiotic. Patients with that kind of problem tend to be poorly: high fever, flushed, achy all over, lacking in energy, and often with a characteristic facial rash and tongue coating.

I looked at my patient. It was difficult to assess his complexion due to the silver face paint blending with the metallic material of his outfit. Nevertheless, he didn't seem too unwell. I checked his temperature – mildly elevated – and established that he also had the typical viral symptom of a runny nose.

'Can you open wide, George?' I said.

Obligingly, he gave me an unobstructed view: big tonsils, with scattered blobs of exudate, but pink rather than angry red. I checked his neck: no real gland swelling.

'I think this one will get better on its own,' I told his mum.

She looked nonplussed. 'But what about the white spots?'

Until a few years ago, no one ever examined their own or their child's tonsils, but these days a complaint of 'white spots' is a common occurrence. It's arisen because of the Centor criteria - a set of four clinical signs devised to help doctors target antibiotic use more appropriately. The presence of tonsillar exudate is one of them, along with a high fever, tender neck glands, and the absence of viral symptoms. If someone scores 4, there's roughly a 50/50 chance that antibiotics might help. Score 2 or less, and it's virtually certain that they won't. The criterion to do with white exudate seems to have taken on a life of its own, though, out there in the big wide world. For many patients/parents it equates to the automatic need for antibiotics.

I explained all this to mum. She seemed satisfied, and took George back to school to enjoy the rest of World Book Day.

Even when a patient scores 4 on the Centor criteria, it remains a moot point whether antibiotics should be used. There's an old medical adage: treat a patient for a sore throat once, and you create a patient for life. In part this is because we teach behaviour: if the doctor thought I needed treatment last time, I'd probably better go back this time. And many doctors, faced with a recurrently consulting patient, simply assume they're demanding antibiotics and go along with it for a quiet life, thereby reinforcing the pattern.

Additionally, by repeatedly treating people, we might actually be preventing their immune system from 'learning' how to mount an effective response to common throat bacteria. Most cases of tonsillitis get better within a week or so, and during that time the immune system develops 'memory' for the infecting germ, so that it rapidly attacks it when it crops up again. Keep killing it off early with antibiotics, and the immune response never properly develops.

The Centor criteria - helpful as they are as a first step in reducing unnecessary antibiotic use – should never supplant clinical judgement. Most Centor 4 cases can safely be allowed to self-limit, but there will be a few where the patient is very unwell and antibiotics are justified. The worst cases of tonsillitis can progress to serious complications, including quinsy – an abscess in the tonsillar bed that can obstruct breathing and swallowing.

As well as reappraising the role for antibiotics, medicine is also increasingly reluctant to perform tonsillectomy. A very small subset of patients, who suffer full-blown tonsillitis multiple times every year, do derive benefit from having their tonsils removed. But an operation that was once routinely performed actually makes very little difference to how often most of us will come down with the next sore throat.

HIGH FIDELITY

CAROL HAD SURVIVED metastatic breast cancer for seven years – far longer than many. Every time her tumour deposits began to escape control from her current treatment, it seemed the oncologists had another trick up their sleeves. She was lucky: each new drug worked brilliantly, knocking the cancer right back, buying her precious more years of life. Sometimes they caused nasty side effects, but it was a price she was more than willing to pay.

She kept working as a PA to a local politician. Petite and gregarious, she loved being in the thick of things, knowing what was going on, chatting to all and sundry about intrigues and issues. She would see me periodically to get repeat prescriptions, or to discuss the latest scan. Always she was upbeat, optimistic. She was aware there could be no cure; that her disease would, at some point, catch up with her. But she would talk about the latest research, about novel drugs coming on-stream. It must have seemed that if she could just keep running, just keep ahead of the cancer, then even more treatment options might become available.

Through all this she was supported by her husband, Ian. Some fifteen years her senior, he was her polar opposite – tall, taciturn, shy. I wondered sometimes what had brought them together, but some pairings just work: she was the bright butterfly; he the sturdy brown stem on which she rested between her gorgeous, fluttering flights.

Eventually, the inevitable happened: a surveillance scan showed disease progression, and the oncologists told her the next drug was the last in the line. Although, like all the rest, it had some effect on the tumour, she began to lose energy. Reluctantly, she gave up her job. I thought this marked the beginning of the end, but she didn't come to see me for some months and I assumed she must be keeping reasonably well.

One of my colleagues brought the news to a coffee-time meeting: Ian had made an appointment to see him, heartbroken that Carol had left. Before long, Carol herself booked into one of my surgeries and turned up with a new man in tow, a tanned chap also around sixty, with a Scouse accent and blond highlights in his shoulder-length hair. Over the coming weeks the story unfolded: Mark was her childhood sweetheart from Liverpool days. They'd reconnected through social media, arranged to meet up, and found that the old chemistry was still there, as strong as ever.

Carol was energised, effervescent. She and Mark did their best to make up for lost time: holidaying in Greece and Turkey, and moving into a flat together. During one appointment, which she attended alone, Carol did express guilt about Ian, but professed herself helpless to do anything other than follow her heart. As a team, our loyalties were painfully divided: it was great to see Carol so full of joy and vigour, but Ian cut a tragic figure, lonely and struggling to rebuild his life following the rejection. Throughout it all, though, he never spoke ill of her to any of us.

In time, the tumour deposits in Carol's chest began to progress. She became permanently breathless, and needed repeated drainage of fluid from around her lungs. Her energy dwindled. Then the news I'd somehow known would come:

Mark was off, back up to Liverpool. The honeymoon, in every sense, was over.

Ian welcomed Carol back to their home. It was one of the most humbling experiences of my career, witnessing the quiet dignity with which he forgave her. Despite the pain she had caused him, he saw the affair for what it was: Carol, finally facing death, coping the only way she knew how, by desperately drinking of life. We talked briefly about it after she'd gone, her liver overwhelmed by the advancing cancer. It was something Ian had come to accept, the price he'd had to pay for sharing his life with a beautiful butterfly. To his eternal credit, he remained faithful to her until the very end.

MUSINGS

LESSONS LEARNED

D AVID WAS A patient during my earliest years in
general practice, an otherwise fit man in his early 60s
who needed an operation on his ear. The procedure went
without a hitch, but afterwards David noticed he was markedly off-balance, and he developed dreadful headaches. His
description stuck in my mind: it was like one side of his skull
was being squeezed and crushed in a vice. He would illustrate
with his hands, clamping and pressing them against his scalp
as he tried to explain.

Initially I hoped it was something that would settle spon-
taneously: side-effects of the general anaesthetic or the painkillers, perhaps; or some deep-seated bruising that would take
a while to resolve. After a few weeks without improvement, I
organised blood tests and examined everything my training
suggested might be relevant. I drew a blank.

My ENT colleagues were similarly perplexed when he attended his six-week follow-up appointment. The surgery had
been successful, they confirmed, and everything was well-
healed. They were at a loss to explain his new symptoms.

So began a tortuous process. The ENT surgeons checked
every angle they could: head scan, x-rays, more bloods, spe-
cialised tests of balance function. Each flurry of activity was
interspersed with interminable periods waiting for the next
outpatient review. Eventually, after many months, the verdict

was delivered: they could find nothing wrong, and could only suggest I refer David to a consultant neurologist instead.

A year later, David was no further forward. He continued to complain bitterly of the grinding headaches, and the dysequilibrium. The neurologist, and an ENT second opinion, had similarly failed to produce a diagnosis. As so often with 'medically unexplained physical symptoms' the spotlight began to shine on the psychosocial sphere: were these symptoms an expression of emotional turmoil? David was emphatic: he had emotional turmoil all right, but it was because that bloody operation had left him crippled and no one seemed to have the first idea how to put him right. His relationship with the medical profession reached rock bottom, and though I tried to support him as best I could, I began to dread seeing his name on my appointment list, so impotent did his case make me feel, and so angry had he become.

Eventually, I moved to another part of the country leaving my first practice, and David's insoluble symptoms, behind. A decade later I myself went in for dental surgery under general anaesthetic. Shortly after getting home I began to feel giddy and off-balance, and I developed headaches that felt like one side of my skull was being crushed in a vice. I tried various measures but nothing helped; weeks went by with no spontaneous improvement. Inevitably, memories of David, and the way his presentation had defeated several specialists, came back to me.

Over the intervening years I had seen a number of perplexing musculoskeletal problems respond to chiropractic treatment where conventional medicine had drawn a blank. I went to discuss my situation with an experienced chiropractor, and he knew immediately what had happened: the surgeon, in manoeuvring my head to get access to the back of my mouth while I was under the anaesthetic, had unwittingly deranged the alignment of the bones at the top of my neck. A few manipulations and my debilitating symptoms simply melted away.

Since learning this lesson I have seen several similar cases where patients can date the onset of back pain or headaches/dizziness to a general anaesthetic. Most doctors are mystified because there's nothing in medical training that teaches that this kind of thing can happen. To a chiropractor, however, it's unsurprising: if you haul insensate bodies from trolleys on to operating tables; if you twist heads this way and that while the protective neck muscles are paralysed by anaesthetic, you will very likely put vertebrae slightly out of kilter, resulting in pain and other dysfunction.

Medicine is a lifelong education. The training we get in our early years is really only a starter guide. Life experiences (our own, and those of family and friends), patients we encounter, stories we hear, continue to expand and refine our understanding of the myriad ways human beings work and don't work. As well as learning lessons from chiropractors, I have also seen startling results on occasions with traditional acupuncture, psychotherapy, even homoeopathy. Yet these kinds of approaches frequently excite derision from conventional doctors, who reject them because they can't be understood in our current scientific terms. If there's one thing that can be said with confidence about our current scientific understanding of the human organism it is that, like all bodies of scientific knowledge, it will be shown in retrospect to have been woefully inadequate over the next 50 years. The provisionality and partiality of our knowledge should serve to keep our minds open and inquisitive to other ways of thinking.

I can now direct a patient with an anaesthetic-related back or neck injury to someone who can help them. My regret is that I didn't have this understanding when David needed help. I can still see him, clamping and pressing his hands to his scalp, trying desperately to communicate what he was going through, but meeting with incomprehension and impotence from his physicians. That has been one of the defining lessons of my career, and I try to remember it whenever a patient presents puzzling problems that defy a conventional diagnostic approach.

MEDICAL MYTHS

F ROM TIME TO time, I remove patients' in-growing
toenails. This is done to help – the condition can be
intractably painful – but it would be barbaric were it not
for anaesthesia. A toe or finger can be rendered completely
numb by a ring block – local anaesthetic injected either side
of the base of the digit, knocking out the nerves that supply
sensation.

The local anaesthetic I use for most surgical procedures
is ready-mixed with adrenaline, which constricts arteries and
thereby reduces bleeding, but ever since medical school I've
had it drummed into me that using adrenaline is a complete
no-no when it comes to ring blocks. The adrenaline cuts off
blood supply to the end of the digit – so the story goes – resulting in tissue death and gangrene. So, prior to performing
any ring block, my practice nurse and I go through an elabo-
rate double-check procedure to ensure that the injection I'm
about to use is 'plain' local anaesthetic with no adrenaline.
This same ritual is observed in hospitals and doctors' surgeries
around the world.

Imagine my surprise, then, to learn recently that this is a
myth. The idea dates back at least a century, to when doctors
frequently found digits turning gangrenous after ring blocks.
The obvious conclusion – that artery-constricting adrenaline
was responsible – still dictates practice to this day. In recent
years, however, the dogma has been questioned. The effect of

adrenaline is partial and short-lived; could it really be causing such catastrophic outcomes?

Retrospective studies of published reports of digital gangrene after ring block identified that adrenaline was actually used in fewer than half the cases. Instead, other factors – including the drastic measures employed to try to prevent infection in the pre-antibiotic era – seemed likely to have been the culprits. Emboldened by these findings, surgeons in America undertook cautious trials to investigate using adrenaline in ring blocks. They found that it caused no tissue damage, and that it made surgery technically easier.

Those ground-breaking trials date back 15 years yet they've only just filtered through, which illustrates how long it takes for new thinking to become disseminated. Currently, a few doctors – mainly in the field of plastic surgery – have changed their practice, but the vast majority of us continue to eschew adrenaline.

Medicine is littered with such myths. For years we doled out antibiotics for minor infections thinking we were speeding recovery and preventing rare serious complications, neither of which has subsequently proved true. Until the mid-1970s, breast cancer was routinely treated with radical mastectomy – a disfiguring operation that removed huge amounts of tissue in the belief that this maximised the chance of cure. These days, we know conservative surgery is at least as effective, and causes vastly less psychological trauma. Seizures can happen in young children with feverish illnesses, so for decades we placed great emphasis on keeping temperatures down. We now know that controlling fever makes no difference, and that the fits are caused not by temperature but by other chemicals released into the circulation during an infection.

Myths arise when the something appears to make complete and obvious sense according to the best understanding we have at the time. In all cases, practice has run far ahead of objective, repeatable science. It is only years after a myth has taken hold that scientific evaluation eventually shows us to have charged off down a blind alley.

Myths, once embedded, are powerful and hard to uproot, even once the science is established. I operated on a toenail just the other week, and still baulked at using adrenaline – partly my own superstition; partly to save my practice nurse from a heart attack. What would it have been like as a pioneering surgeon in the 1970s, treating breast cancer with a simple lumpectomy while the bulk of your colleagues believed you were being reckless with your patients' future health? Decades of dire warnings and established practice create a hefty weight to overturn. Only once a good proportion of the medical herd has changed course do most of us feel confident to follow suit.

PAIN

RARE INDIVIDUALS BORN without pain perception (congenital insensitivity to pain, CIP) rapidly accumulate disabilities, and tend to die young. Pain makes us withdraw from and subsequently avoid injurious situations, it prompts us to protect damaged structures such as eyes or joints, and it alerts us to diseases such as appendicitis that without treatment may prove fatal. And what is true of physical pain is also true of its emotional counterpart. Pain is good for us. It helps us to survive.

But what if pain perception goes haywire? Like all UK general practitioners I have several patients with a frustrating if fascinating condition called fibromyalgia. Jane is typical of the severe end of the spectrum: she's a woman in her 40s (early middle-aged women are most frequently affected), her life is blighted by unremitting pain in muscles throughout her body, and no painkiller gives her any relief (she has tried them all, even morphine). Over the years she's become progressively disabled, finding it harder to do even simple things like help her young children dress, and able to work fewer and fewer hours. Around 18 months ago she went long-term sick, and earlier this year her employer terminated her contract. She's now struggling to adjust to a life on benefits. Apart from the constant pain, one of the things she worries about most is other people's disbelief. To casual observation, Jane appears in the pink of health.

People with fibromyalgia have precious little to show for their suffering. They have no swelling, inflammation, limp, or deformity. Blood tests, X-rays, scans, and biopsies are normal. Theirs is a subjective illness. They find that family and friends eventually tire of hearing about their intractable pain and its impacts. Little wonder that depression and anxiety are common complications. To cap it all, their doctors frequently grow frustrated as they return, time and again, to report a distinct lack of improvement with each and every treatment that's tried. Over the years, many physicians have questioned fibromyalgia's validity as a disease; physical symptoms are dismissed as 'all in the mind', the implication being that, in an unconscious way, these patients 'need' their illness as a passport to duck out from the stresses and strains and dissat-isfactions of everyday life.

Advances in imaging the functioning nervous system are beginning to shed light on what's really going on. To experience pain, you have to have the requisite sensory apparatus: receptors (nociceptors) that detect harmful changes within the body's tissues and organs; and nerve cells (neurones) that relay this in-formation to the brain. It's this sensory apparatus that's missing in those rare individuals with CIP. But sensing alone is not enough. Once pain nerve signals reach the brain they are subject to what is termed central processing, involving a number of the brain's most evolutionarily primitive regions, regions that are involved with raw emotional response – with fight, flight and survival. It's this central processing that transforms nociceptor sensory input into our subjective experience of pain.

There's a heck of a lot of other nerve traffic passing from body to brain that's got nothing to do with pain. For example, our muscles are constantly generating information as to their position, stretch, and contraction, all of which ensures the apparently effortless coordination of our movements and balance. In fibromyalgia, some of this non-pain information seems to become capable of triggering the brain's central pain processing regions. The very fact of having normally functioning muscles begins to be experienced as chronic, widespread pain.

It's not fully clear what causes this malfunction, but a process called central sensitisation is at its heart. We know that 30% of patients with uncontrolled rheumatoid arthritis – where diseased joints constantly bombard the brain with nociceptive input – will eventually develop superimposed fibromyalgia. Sheer volume of pain traffic in the nervous system may be one factor in central sensitisation.

However, many fibromyalgia sufferers don't have a pre-existing painful arthritis. Their fibromyalgia may be linked to genetically disposed abnormalities in brain chemistry. The chemicals (neurotransmitters) involved in central pain processing have different functions elsewhere in the nervous system, which may account for the additional symptoms many fibromyalgia patients experience – sleep disturbance, profound fatigue, and impaired concentration and thinking ('fibrofog'). What causes these neurotransmitter abnormalities to be 'unmasked' at a certain time – resulting in fibromyalgia – is as yet unclear, but intriguing studies into 'pain memory' suggest that stresses in adult life may reignite central sensitisation originally developed in the context of severe emotional or physical pain when young, something that may explain the association between fibromyalgia and childhood abuse or trauma.

We're still a long way from understanding fibromyalgia and treating it effectively, but we are at least now aware that, as an illness, it's all in the brain, if not the mind.

LLOYD GEORGE

I N THE EARLY decades of the NHS, medical records were filed in what are called Lloyd George envelopes – a folder 5x7 inches in size, made of stiff manilla card, and able to expand to about 2 inches' thickness for those occasional patients who had large numbers of letters and lab reports. The envelopes' design dates back to the early 20th century. They were named after David Lloyd George, the Liberal Chancellor and later Prime Minister, and were used in the National Insurance 'panel system' he instituted in 1911, an early attempt at socially funded healthcare in Britain, and a forerunner of the NHS.

By the time I entered practice in the 1990s, Lloyd George envelopes had become unfit for purpose. Our increasingly litigious culture meant notes had become copious, several paragraphs being written where once a doctor might simply have recorded a diagnosis and treatment. And the burgeoning capacity of modern medicine to *do* things meant having to cram in ever more test results, radiology reports, and correspondence between GPs and specialists. The envelopes bulged to bursting, and even though reception staff became adept at 'extending' them, the contents were frequently unmanageable, letters and reports becoming creased and torn as they were extracted, unfolded, read, and squashed back in.

In 2000, a variation was made to NHS legislation to allow doctors to hold medical records on computer instead, and this has rapidly become the norm. The old Lloyd George envelopes are still with us – every NHS patient is required to have one – but these days they gather dust on racks of shelving in GP surgeries, rarely if ever consulted, anachronistic in our digitised, 'big data' era.

The only time I look through one is when an insurance company commissions a medical report, and I need to delve back into a patient's distant past history. Currently, these tend to be for people born in the 1960s, 70s, and 80s. GP records then were handwritten, pithy, and sometimes barely legible. They were never signed, but the pages of identical script speaks of the continuous care provided by one or two doctors over years or even decades. There were remarkably few drugs available to treat illnesses – a doctor would have held a working knowledge of the entire pharmacopoeia in their head, something that is now utterly impossible.

Letters between GPs and consultants read like historical documents: formal and courteous, succinctly phrased, typed out and carbon-copied on manual typewriters. They illustrate how much has changed over the course of these patients' lifetimes. Childhood operations like tonsillectomy, or inserting grommets for glue ear, used to be performed at the drop of a hat. These days they have fallen out of favour, partly as evidence has emerged of their relative ineffectiveness, partly as a result of the NHS's relentless cost-containment drive.

Every now and again, the Lloyd George envelope I'm reading belongs to a troubled adult: patients with personality disorders, or uncontrolled addictions, or those whose lives have disintegrated through repeated relationship and career breakdowns. Buried in the correspondence in their Lloyd George envelopes, one often finds the same patterns and clues.

Back in the 1960s and 70s, 'difficult' children would be seen in what were called 'child guidance clinics'. Letters from their psychiatrists talk of 'delinquency' and discuss the challenges posed by their problematic behaviours. There was some insight into the way parents and families might affect a developing child, but the main focus of therapy was on the children themselves and how to overcome their apparent neuroses in order to get them to behave more acceptably. It was definitely the child who had the problem; definitely the child who needed the 'guidance'.

I know these patients as adults, and am familiar with the stories of childhood abuse – physical, emotional, sexual – that they have latterly been able to tell. Looked at from this vantage point, the child guidance clinic letters read tragically – it never appears to have crossed anyone's mind what these 'difficult' children might actually have been experiencing. And indeed it wouldn't have. Reading the standard child guidance textbooks from the 1970s, one finds no discussion of the possibility that adults, most often parents, could be inflicting horrific abuse. Today we understand that 'a difficult child is a child in difficulty'. A generation ago, the understanding of those difficulties was wholly inadequate, founded on a belief that almost all parents were fundamentally decent adults who wanted the best for their offspring, and blinkered by a collective ignorance of what might be going on behind closed doors.

These cases come to mind when I hear media reports about historic abuse cases going through the courts. How, it is often asked, could now-convicted perpetrators have been able to get away with their offences for so long – sometimes continuing to offend even after reassuring police, social workers, employers, or others in authority of the baselessness of contemporaneous allegations? The answer, in part, lies in the sheaves of correspondence filed in those rows of Lloyd George envelopes. The world they depict was a much simpler, more innocent one – or at least that was how it seemed to professionals of the time. These days we have a harsher comprehension of what some people are capable of, and the damage they propagate as a result. Hopefully the next generation, whose own Lloyd George envelopes are destined to remain empty and anachronistic, will be better protected and served.

FAT TAX

WITHIN THE LAST few years, we've reached the milestone of two thirds of the adult population being either overweight (body mass index over 25) or obese (BMI over 30). The statistic reminded me of another I've come across recently: that in the 1960s, the period we now recognise as the peak of the UK smoking epidemic, fully 70% of men and 40% of women were smokers.

At such levels of prevalence, cultural perceptions alter. It appears normal for people to smoke, a conclusion subliminally supported by the ready availability of tobacco; by the provision of paraphernalia such as ashtrays in planes, trains, and cars; and by adverts in every form of media. We are currently witnessing a similar 'normalisation' of obesity, with shop mannequins getting larger, 'inflation' in clothing sizes (when is a size 10 no longer a size 10?), and furniture design altering to accommodate the new norms.

The historic smoking prevalence data stands in stark contrast to he present day picture: the proportion of smokers in the English population has fallen below 20% for the first time. And the campaign waged against tobacco over the past 50 years tells us everything we need to know about effecting a similar reduction in rates of obesity.

The prerequisite is information. The tide started to turn against smoking following the publication, in 1962, of the first study to demonstrate an unequivocal link with lung cancer.

The drip-drip of new health information gathered pace and by the 1970s the hitherto inexorable rise in smoking prevalence began to reverse. The strong links between obesity and conditions such as heart disease, stroke, diabetes, and three of the four commonest cancers (bowel, breast and prostate) are well-established, but have yet to lodge in the public consciousness. Most people are aware that being substantially overweight is somehow not good for you, but have only a vague idea as to the true extent of the problem. I have several obese patients who have been shocked to learn that their weight poses comparable risks of disability and premature death as if they were inveterate smokers.

Information alone is insufficient. Losing weight is, for most people, at least as challenging as quitting nicotine, and research is making clear that large 'hits' of sugar – be it 'off the spoon', or 'hidden' in processed foodstuffs – have addictive potential. The same may also be true of fried foods. The NHS is gradually waking up to the need to provide structured support to people keen to lose weight, in much the same way as it devotes considerable resources to smoking cessation services.

These sorts of approaches harness people's sense of personal responsibility, but experience of tackling smoking suggests that wider measures will also be needed. Stiff taxation has made smoking much less affordable, driving down demand. Advertising and shop display prohibition, and obligatory stark health warnings on packaging, have contributed to the message that tobacco use is no longer normal behaviour. Bans on smoking in public places – and in cars with children – intended to protect against passive smoking, also serve to marginalise smoking further.

The situation is more complex for obesity. Eating and

drinking are normal activities, and there is no single culprit product on which government can train its sights. Having said that, there's good evidence on which ministers could get to work. Sugar in soft drinks, and added almost routinely to processed foods, makes a major contribution to overall calorie intake. There should be an immediate ban on any product being marketed as 'low' or 'no fat' – or, indeed, trumpeting its freedom from 'artificial flavourings and additives' – when it is stuffed full of sugar instead (as most are). Breakfast cereals, particularly those aimed at children, are, by and large, a national scandal. Several European countries have already introduced a 'sugar tax' and the UK should follow suit, though the sugar industry, as the tobacco industry before it, will resist with vigorous lobbying.

The junk food industry is also under the spotlight. A neat piece of research published recently in the *British Medical Journal* established clear links between obesity rates and the density of fast-food outlets around people's homes, workplaces, and along their commuting routes. Will there come a time when diners consuming reasonably priced, healthy wholefoods sit comfortably inside warm restaurants, while shame-faced burger-munchers huddle beneath a shelter in the windswept car park bemoaning the punitive taxes levied on their fast-food fix?

In our efforts to tackle the obesity epidemic, care is needed not to stigmatise the overweight. A small proportion of obesity is genetically determined. For the rest, outward appearances are rarely indicative of simplistic so-called failings such as gluttony. Excess weight is driven by the low-cost energy-dense foodstuffs ubiquitously arrayed around us, by the time- and exercise-poor lifestyles our culture currently demands, and by a failure of education and information to keep pace with the rapid changes that food technology has wrought over the past four decades. Obesity can also be a manifestation of the same emotional wounds that drive more conventional addictions. We need compassion on ourselves and on each other. But as the smoking epidemic smoulders towards its conclusion, we need to face up to the public health crisis that has grown in its wake, and we need to shape up fast.

This column was originally published in 2014. In 2018 the UK government introduced a 'sugar tax' on highly calorific soft drinks. London has introduced a ban on junk food advertising on buses and the tube.

MOBILE MEDICINE

M Y SENIOR PARTNER can remember his wife being
stuck indoors whenever he was on call, in order to
answer the phone. She would have his itinerary, and would
ring round various patients' homes to track him down when
a new visit needed adding to the list, or if something urgent
had cropped up.

Pagers were the norm by the time I started, though one
still had to find a phone to return a message when out and
about. Before long, though, our practice acquired one of the
new mobile telephones (not quite brick-sized, but not far off)
and we were never out of contact again – as long as there was
signal, of course.

These days, virtually everyone has a mobile so patients
are instantly reachable, too. This has transformed telephone
consulting: many discussions can be handled without someone
having to trek to the surgery for an appointment, or to stay
glued to their landline waiting for the doctor's call. Signal is
still frustratingly variable in our semi-rural area: conversations have a habit of hanging at crucial points, and distor-
tion can sometimes make it sound like I'm consulting with
a Dalek.

One gets used to catching people at awkward moments.
I've spoken to several who have confessed that they're on the
loo. And the more embarrassing the problem the more likely
it is the patient will be in the midst of some meeting or social

gathering: it can take ages to extricate themselves to ensure the necessary privacy.

Ultra-availability occasionally creates interesting scenarios. I recently had a message to ring Tina. Tina suffers from hypomania and if one happens to get her when unwell it can tie up a huge amount of time, so I was a bit apprehensive dialling her mobile number. Sure enough, she was very obviously high – I could scarcely get a word in edgeways as she regaled me with all sorts of disjointed and irrational experiences. I kept trying to find out where she actually was – she was clearly very unwell and was going to need assessment. Eventually, after 25 minutes of hypomanic monologue I managed to establish that I was ringing her in a psychiatric ward on the other side of the country where she was currently detained under a Mental Health Act section. At least there was nothing I had to do.

The rise of the smartphone has augmented mere availability. Both doctors and patients can access limitless medical information at the drop of a hat. Apps remind people to take medication, send orders for repeat prescriptions, and can monitor vital signs such as heart rate and rhythm, and blood oxygen levels. These will only get more sophisticated.

The most impressive app I've so far encountered belongs to a Polish patient who speaks about three words of English: a voice-recognition, auto-transcribing Polish-English translation engine. We have conducted several consultations to date, handing his phone back and forth between us. It's uncanny, watching it turn my speech into text – you can actually see it altering words between homophones as it correctly re-interprets the context. Then at the touch of the screen my sentences are rendered in both audio and written Polish, and his vice versa.

It's astonishingly accurate. The only glitch was when he tried to tell me that, at 67 years old, he's started to have problems with his dad. I wasn't surprised: his father was probably a nonagenarian. I tried to find out the nature of the difficulties: was it dementia, or advancing frailty with all its attendant care needs? It took several puzzling exchanges before the penny dropped. 'Dad' turns out to be an unfortunate mistranslation of a Polish euphemism for the male member. I've since been able to help the prostate problems that were making it increasingly difficult to pee.

The huge leap in technology in the space of a single generation has led to speculation that smartphones and apps will gradually displace doctors. I don't doubt we'll see further amazing advances, but medicine is an intensely human, interpersonal art. Technology will assist, but it won't replace us. And, in any case, we would need to sort out the signal first.

IN HOURS

KYLIE AND THE RASH

DANNY'S RASH HAD no diagnostic features, so I suggested running some blood tests to try to work out what was going on. He appeared worried that it hadn't proved straightforward.

'Where do think it's come from, then?' he asked.

His choice of words tweaked my antennae. Usually a patient will ask, 'What do you think's causing it?' or 'Am I allergic to something?'

'You're worried about where it's come from?' I echoed back.

Danny paused for a second, as though weighing up what to say.

'It was after a Kylie concert, down in London,' he told me, his voice rueful. He rolled his eyes in a pantomime of What-am-I-like? '*Such* a gay thing to do.'

'You're concerned this might be HIV?'

He nodded, his expression glum now that his underlying fear had been articulated.

People exposed to HIV often undergo a seroconversion illness 2 - 6 weeks later as the virus takes hold. A rash can be a feature. Danny told me his skin had first flared a few weeks after the Kylie-concert encounter. Although the timing was suggestive, I didn't think HIV was likely. His rash was itchy, for one thing; and it had persisted for some time. So I made reassuring noises, but offered to add an HIV test to the investigations. I asked him to book a follow-up appointment:

it's never a good idea to find yourself discussing potentially difficult news on the phone.

The HIV test came back negative, but among the other results was a big surprise. I'd checked Danny's iron levels – iron deficiency is a frequent cause of skin itch. Far from being deficient, however, Danny was super-saturated. There's really only one explanation for such a picture – a disease called haemochromatosis – but as far as I was aware, this condition didn't cause a rash. A couple of minutes later, though, and Google had turned up two reports in the medical literature of rare cases presenting exactly as Danny's had done.

For most of us, iron is poorly absorbed from food; the small amount we extract roughly balances the daily losses through normal bodily function. People with haemochromatosis, however, are abnormally efficient at absorbing dietary iron, and because the excess cannot be excreted, over decades they accumulate vast stores. Eventually, the inexorable deposition of iron begins to damage their tissues, causing liver cirrhosis and cancer, and heart failure. The treatment sounds medieval but it's effective: sufferers undergo frequent blood-letting – a pint every week in the early phases of therapy – in order to leach the iron back out.

Haemochromatosis is the commonest single gene disorder in Northern Europe: around 1 in 200 Caucasian people are genetically susceptible. Progression to clinical haemochromatosis happens much less frequently than this, though. It's unusual for women to develop the condition – the menstrual cycle helps prevent iron reaching toxic levels – and anyone who regularly donates blood is also unknowingly protecting themselves. Variations in diet, together with subtle interplays

with other relevant genes, probably keep many other susceptible people from developing the disease.

These days, genetic tests also allow screening of individuals with a positive family history. If confirmed as genetically
vulnerable, they can be monitored, and treatment commenced
well before any organ damage occurs. There was no apparent
history in Danny's family, though. Discussing things at his
follow-up appointment it became clear why: Danny revealed
that he'd been adopted as a baby, and nothing was known of
his birth parents.

I sent him to a specialist for a liver biopsy. The news was
excellent: no sign of scarring or cirrhosis. A crash course
of blood-letting brought his iron levels gradually lower, and
maintenance bleeds will keep him out of trouble long-term.
The origin of his condition lay in a family he knew nothing
about. Fortunately for him, his fear that it had originated
one night after a Kylie concert prompted him to seek medical
advice that, quite by chance, established the true diagnosis
while there was still time to do something about it.

COMPLAINT

VERONICA CAME TO see me on an urgent appointment. She was extremely anxious, convinced there must be something seriously wrong with her heart. She'd had pain in her chest for a couple of days, but hadn't thought too much about it until she'd mentioned it to her boss that morning. Veronica happens to work as a secretary for a consultant surgeon. He'd appeared concerned, and had immediately phoned a cardiology colleague. Much to Veronica's consternation, she was told to go straight to her GP to get blood tests and an ECG.

It didn't take me long to establish the diagnosis – she was exquisitely tender over the joints at the ends of the ribs, a condition called costochondritis. It gets better with time and judicious ibuprofen. There certainly wasn't anything wrong with her heart, and she definitely didn't need any tests. I passed on the good news, wished her a speedy recovery, and cracked on with the last patients of the morning.

The following week, my practice manager presented me with Veronica's letter of complaint. In it, she described how I'd made her feel 'stupid' for coming to see me. My initial reaction was of surprise, shock even; and an abrupt sense of defensiveness. I replayed the consultation in my mind. How on earth could she have misinterpreted it as me thinking she was 'stupid'?

Written complaints against doctors were infrequent when

I started in practice in the early 1990s; now, the average GP expects at least one a year. This almost certainly reflects an increased readiness to complain across our society, rather than a decline in medical care or communication. Medical complaints are best understood in terms of four domains – the patient, the illness, the system, and the doctor – all of which play a part in virtually every contentious scenario.

Being human, I found it easy enough to identify the issues with the first three. Veronica was highly anxious when she consulted, which may have distorted her perceptions. As for her illness, although ultimately it proved to be something trivial, its cardinal symptom – chest pain – often leads it to be confused with serious pathology. The system was also contributory. Veronica wasn't 'officially' a patient of the cardiologist, so he'd obtained just enough information to decide she didn't constitute an emergency, then had sent her off in my direction for a proper evaluation. He would never consult a cardiological patient without an ECG and routine blood tests beforehand; and he has no experience of general practice to appreciate that we perform investigations much more selectively.

Being human, I found it uncomfortable to confront the issues with the fourth domain: the doctor. Yet this is the only one over which I have any real influence. The acronym, HALT, is useful: hungry, angry, late, tired. Veronica's emergency appointment had been tacked on the end of a long surgery that was, by then, running very late, with all the stress that causes. I'd consulted 18 other patients before her, and it was getting near to lunch, so I was both fatigued and ravenous. As for anger, we all have our particular 'hot buttons' – those things that instantly infuriate us. I remembered the irritation I'd felt at the cardiologist blithely instructing that I do various investigations that were completely pointless, treating me like a junior house officer and heightening my patient's anxiety in the process.

At the time, I'd tried to explain to Veronica why she didn't need the tests she'd been told she should have. Being hungry, late, and tired, I evidently didn't handle my annoyance with the cardiologist well. It must have been apparent though, if not in my words then in my body language and tone of voice. Veronica perceived this as my being irritated with her, making her feel 'stupid' for coming.

I sent her a letter of apology. Veronica's costochondritis quickly settled. And I learned lessons that might help me manage a similar situation more adroitly in the future.

AUBREY

A FEW MONTHS earlier, Brenda had been diagnosed with Parkinson's disease, but the nebulous back pain that prompted the home visit request wasn't a result of that. As I asked more about her symptoms, I became conscious of an air of bewilderment about her. I started to wonder whether depression – common after any significant diagnosis, and often a feature of Parkinson's – might be part of the picture.

Throughout the discussion her husband, Aubrey, stood awkwardly off to one side, in a no-man's-land midway between her chair and the doorway, as though unsure whether to stay in the room or leave it. He made a couple of brief contributions, but in the main he just listened. When I asked Brenda whether she was still enjoying the things she usually loved in life, she turned to him and – somewhat accusingly – commented that they rarely went away any more. I could sense something between them, some issue, but I didn't know what it was.

Aubrey came to see me in surgery soon afterwards. He'd found a lovely convalescent home, he told me, and he wanted to take Brenda there for a six-week break. The thing was, he needed me to complete a health form for them. I scanned the document: I had no idea there was such a thing as a convalescent home still in existence – the idea seemed quaint, Victorian. But there it was: on the front of the pamphlet was a line drawing of an old manor house in the Home Counties that now served as a sort of genteel hotel-with-nurses.

Leave it with me, I told him. I was touched by the way he'd responded to Brenda's complaint about her restricted life, and impressed that he'd managed to find such a splendid-looking retreat. By the way, he said, wincing as he stood up to go, I've been suffering with some of that backache, too, you know.

Aubrey's back pain, in contrast to his wife's, worried me: new in onset and with no cause, affecting the upper spine, worse when lying down, waking him from sleep. An urgent MRI revealed advanced lung cancer eroding his vertebrae. At some point while waiting for the scan results, I did fill in the convalescent home forms for him, but he and Brenda never got to go. Over the next five weeks he declined rapidly, and died peacefully at home.

Their daughter, Jill, rallied round during the crisis, but had to pick her normal life back up after Aubrey died. Problems quickly became apparent. Brenda's meals generally didn't happen unless prepared for her and supervised, and she frequently forgot to take her Parkinson's medication, or else took the various sets of pills laid out for the whole day all in one go. Then there were the evening phone calls: Brenda ringing Jill repeatedly, distraught about the faceless people sitting in the chairs in her lounge, or loitering in her hallway.

We arranged emergency respite care while the true picture emerged. Rather than 'pure' Parkinson's disease – which affects a brain region principally concerned with movement, the substantia nigra – Brenda was suffering from Lewy body disease. This often presents like Parkinson's initially, the substantia nigra being an early casualty of the degenerative changes. But within months, other areas of the brain begin to be affected, producing a pattern of dementia that's quite distinct from more common forms such as Alzheimer's. The visual cortex is frequently involved, and around three-quarters of Lewy body sufferers experience marked visual hallucinations. Brenda's brain was misperceiving the coats on the pegs, and the anti-macassars on the armchairs, and turning them into grotesque, featureless-faced people that she alone could see.

Although Lewy body disease develops more rapidly than other types of dementia, the degree of difficulty Brenda was experiencing did not come on overnight. When I talked about it with Jill, it made perfect sense for her of several incidents over the preceding months. It became apparent that Aubrey had been coping with, and covering up, his wife's symptoms for some time.

Spouses frequently 'compensate' for their partner's demen-tia for considerable periods without involving professionals. The reasons are complex and have to do with denial, with fear, with shame, with loyalty, and with stoicism. Not infre-quently a dementia diagnosis is apparent only when something happens to destabilise the situation – a hospital admission, or the spouse's untimely death. I think back to that home visit: Brenda with her nebulous back pain, Aubrey wavering between her chair and the sitting room door. I sensed indeci-sion in him. How long had he been coping with her distressing evening hallucinations, organising her meals and medication, keeping the outside world at bay? It must have taken a toll. Was he fearful that she might let slip something that would reveal the extent of her problems? Or was he secretly hoping that might happen, a way for him to get help without the guilt of admitting he needed it?

That six-week break stays in my mind. I remember think-ing a convalescent home was a bit over-the-top; they would have been fine in a regular hotel. Aubrey knew better though, and I admire him for it. Brenda's disturbing visual hallucinations and fluctuating confusion meant having nurses on hand would have been reassuring. He'd organised the perfect holiday, and I only wish they'd got to enjoy it.

THE SKIN WE'RE IN

ROBBIE HAD HAD a sore throat and fluey symptoms, and the large patch of inflamed skin that appeared on one side of his abdomen hadn't particularly bothered him, especially as it started to fade when he began to feel better. That morning, though, he'd woken to find himself covered in dozens of similar patches scattered all over his body.

He looked worried. Dermatological diseases aren't often serious, but they can cause distressing symptoms such as itch, and they almost invariably impact on our psychology. Our skin is our interface with the world. When something goes wrong with it, it can create embarrassment and even shame – ancient notions of uncleanliness, sinfulness and contagion persist to this day. Robbie was in his early twenties; he wanted to be out playing the mating game. Were he to disrobe in front of a prospective partner looking like this, they'd run a mile.

I asked a few questions as he unbuttoned his shirt. Two of the commonest dermatological conditions we see – eczema and psoriasis – have variants that might have fitted the bill, but they tend to run in families, and Robbie had no affected relatives. One of my other hunches was confirmed as soon as I saw the rash. Lines of oval pinky-red patches swept symmetrically across his trunk in gentle curves reminiscent of the branches of a Christmas tree.

'It's something called pityriasis rosea,' I explained. The virus that had made him feel poorly also affects the skin. It starts with a single 'herald patch', just as Robbie had noticed, followed a week or two later by a dramatic outbreak of secondary lesions. These tend to be flat and salmon pink, and often have a ruff of fine scales around their edges. Robbie's rash lacked this last feature; then again, it's rare to see textbook cases of anything.

Dermatology is one of the branches of medicine Sherlock Holmes would have most relished were he, like Watson, to have become a doctor. There are hundreds of different rashes and each has tell-tale, though often subtle signs that, with careful observation, can lead clinicians to the correct diagnosis.

One of the most intriguing features of rashes is that they tend to have characteristic distributions. Coxsackie virus typically affects the extremities and the oral area, hence its colloquial name, 'hand, foot and mouth disease'. Parvovirus homes in on the sides of the face; it's known as 'slapped cheek syndrome'. The many different patterns of eczema also affect particular areas: atopic eczema inflames the fronts of the elbows and behind the knees; seborrhoeic eczema presents along the sides of the nose, the eyebrows, and the front of the chin. An intensely itchy condition, lichen planus, has a predilection for the wrists, where it has a violet hue, and the insides of the cheeks where it forms lacy white webs.

In a few instances, we understand why these characteristic distributions occur. Shingles, caused by reactivation of the chickenpox virus, reaches the skin by travelling along a single nerve: this results a one-sided rash confined to the area – known as a dermatome – supplied by the affected nerve. The virus that caused Robbie's pityriasis probably migrates in a similar way, though its 'Christmas tree' distribution maps multiple dermatomes on both sides of the body.

For the most part, though, we have no idea why different rashes affect certain areas of skin and not others. With enough research we could doubtless develop some fascinating insights. However, it is unlikely this would enhance treatment, so such research will probably never be funded. I rather like the mystery of it all – it's as though nature is playing us, dropping us little clues to help us make our diagnoses.

Many rashes we can do nothing about, but at least with the right diagnosis I could tell Robbie what to expect. He was pleased to hear his pityriasis would eventually get better, but dismayed to learn that it could take a few months and there was nothing we could do to hurry the process along. As he got up to leave, I sensed he'd resigned himself to an enforced pause in the mating game.

TEXTBOOK STUFF

MARY, MY REGISTRAR, had been consulted by Jake, a quarryman in his mid-thirties, who was complaining of feeling unaccountably weak. As presenting symptoms go that's pretty non-specific, and could have been a feature of innumerable conditions. His vague tummy aches, occasional nausea, and unintentional weight loss didn't help narrow it down much, either. But the whole picture had been sufficiently concerning for Mary to have arranged some blood tests.

'Look what's come back on his electrolytes,' she said to me.

I peered at the results on her screen. Sodium level well below normal; potassium level a touch high.

'I wondered about Addison's. But it can't be, can it?'

I understood her disbelief. Addison's disease – which sees destruction of the adrenal glands, where the steroid hormone cortisol is made – is so rare that a UK GP will encounter a new case only once in their entire career, if at all. And if they do come across one, they'll likely miss it. Addison's is notorious for giving rise to vague, non-specific symptoms, which get put down to virtually anything else. The majority of Addison's patients end up seeing a succession of doctors before someone at last twigs what's going on. The average delay between first presentation and eventual diagnosis is two years. For Mary to have sorted a case in one consultation would be quite something.

'Check his cortisol,' I said. 'That'll settle it.'

Sure enough, a couple of days later Jake's cortisol level came back from the lab, abnormally low.

'Well done,' I told Mary. 'That was a great spot.'

She's a very modest person, and made some noises about it having been a textbook case. Most Addison's in the UK is caused by an aberrant immune system, which mistakenly attacks the adrenal gland tissue. As such, it is often associated with other autoimmune conditions, and Mary mentioned that Jake had also proved to have vitiligo – scattered patches of lily-white skin where the pigment cells have been destroyed by an abnormal immune response.

'Text book or not,' I said, 'you got on top of it straight away. You've done Jake a huge service.'

Addison's is infamous for causing disasters. Cortisol plays a vital role in the body's response to infection, and undiagnosed Addison's patients can quickly die from what in anyone else would be a trivial illness such as gastroenteritis. The medical literature – and not infrequently the law courts – periodically deal with cases where Addison's has only been discovered at post-mortem. Devastating for the patient and their family, and awful too for the doctors who, in retrospect, realise what it was they'd been missing. Jake will be able to live a normal life now, his energy restored by daily hormone tablets, and his cupboard stocked with a cortisone injection to give himself in the event that he becomes acutely unwell.

Mary's triumph set me thinking about Iain, a printer in his late twenties who'd been consulting me for six months with baffling leg weakness. His symptoms had gradually pro-gressed such that he was now unable to stand for more than a couple of hours before being completely wiped out. Among innumerable tests, I'd checked his electrolytes and they'd come back normal. Then again, the characteristic pattern of derangement that Mary had picked up in Jake is absent in at least a fifth of Addison's cases, so I hadn't ruled it out. And Iain had both vitiligo and autoimmune thyroid disease. But. Mary diagnosing Addison's was a rare enough event – surely two doctors in one practice could never pull off the same feat in the space of a week?

My instinctive doubtfulness reminded me of Mary's initial reaction when faced with Jake's results – and everything about Iain's case now seemed to scream *Addison's!* at me. I called him and arranged a cortisol the following morning, increasingly excited that I might soon have the answer to his mysterious illness.

The result came back plumb normal, completely ruling out Addison's. I'm back to square one with Iain's failing limbs. Sometimes medicine goes according to the text books. Many more times, it does not.

The solution to Iain's problems turned out to be his underactive thyroid. Despite his blood tests indicating that his thyroid hormone replacement was at the right dose, the range of 'normal' values for that blood test is actually quite wide. We discovered that his symptoms completely resolved with a slightly higher dose of thyroid hormone; his blood test remained within the 'normal range' but just a lot higher up it than it had been. Just as not all abnormal medical test results are truly abnormal, not all normal readings are normal either.

LOST HOURS

A WEEK BEFORE, Graham had suffered a head injury. He'd sustained a sizeable laceration at the back of his scalp, and the impact must have been of sufficient force to knock him out cold. He could remember leaving his brother's 40th birthday celebrations at about one in the morning. His next memory was of being in A&E having his wound stitched. He'd been told that a passer-by had found him wondering aimlessly, covered in blood, and had summoned an ambulance, but he had no recollection of these events at all.

A period of amnesia is invariable with a significant brain injury, and indeed it serves as a gauge of severity. In the worst cases, whole weeks or months of life can be irretrievably lost. Graham had a gap of a couple of hours, meaning his outlook was good: full recovery could be expected. Nevertheless, the post-concussion symptoms he was experiencing – headaches, dizzy spells, irritability, and poor concentration – were likely to persist for up to six weeks. The brain is cushioned inside the protective case of the skull by a bath of cerebrospinal fluid (CSF). CSF absorbs the shocks of day-to-day activities, but is unable fully to mitigate the effects of powerful deceleration forces. Post-concussion syndrome can be thought of as the gradual resolution of the bruising and swelling of the brain that arises in such circumstances.

One immediate problem was knowing what had caused the injury. Graham had been more than merry when he left the party to walk home, so the likeliest thing was a slip or stumble causing him to fall backwards and crack his head on the pavement. Other explanations were possible, though: he could have had a seizure, for instance, or perhaps suffered a disturbance of heart rhythm causing him to faint and fall. Being a previously healthy father-of-three in his late thirties meant these were unlikely, but not impossible. The lack of an eyewitness, together with Graham's amnesia, meant we were never going to know. The only thing was to wait and see: if there had been an underlying problem then it would very likely recur.

He returned the following week with a new air of bewilderment about him. He said he wanted to discuss 'the assault'. In the days since I'd seen him, the police had been in contact to say his bag – missing since the incident – had been found abandoned in a front garden. His wallet had been stripped of cash and credit cards. Most disturbingly, evidence of his blood had been found at shoulder-height on a nearby wall. The police's inference was that he'd been shoved hard into the brickwork, sustaining the knock-out blow. His assailant(s) had then taken everything of value in his bag, leaving him unconscious in the street.

People come to terms with traumatic events in different ways, but memory is a crucial common factor. We replay things again and again in our minds over a prolonged period, gradually processing and moving on from what has happened. For some, the emotions aroused are intolerable: memories are repressed instead and the trauma remains unprocessed, its effects resurfacing in nightmares and flashbacks and the myriad other psychological symptoms that comprise post-traumatic stress disorder (PTSD).

For Graham, the challenge was different – he had no memory either to process or repress. He would probably never know who had attacked him, what had actually gone on between them, whether he could have done anything to avoid it happening. Indeed, while the police's account sounded plausible, he would probably always be dogged by uncertainty as to whether it was the truth.

Gently, I encouraged him to get back to work and return to normal life. The greatest threat to him now was to become 'stuck' in his presumed victimhood. The greatest protection against that lay in re-immersing himself in family, friendships, and the other roles that had given him his sense of self prior to the night of the lost hours.

BLUE BOOK

ETHAN'S PARENTS HAD already had one health scare: a heart murmur, picked up shortly after he was born. But it hadn't turned out to be serious: a modest narrowing of the artery taking blood from heart to lungs. Ethan was under hospital follow-up, but no one seemed to think it would need surgical intervention.

Now this. 'The health visitor said to bring him,' Ethan's mum explained. 'He's late with his smile.'

Milly handed me Ethan's 'red book'. This is the parent-held health record, named for its bright red plastic cover, which contains all the information about a child's growth and development. I leafed through the notes from his 6-week check. Most babies have developed a social smile by that age. Ethan hadn't, so he'd been monitored. He was now 4 months, and still no sign of smiling. The health visitor had also noted concerns about head control.

I turned to look at him, cradled in Milly's arms. He was alert, eyes fixed on the beaded rope that attached his dummy to his baby-gro. One hand was reaching out, making erratic contact with the smooth white beads. His developing brain was hard at it, organising visual, spatial and tactile information into an evolving model of the world. This was reassuringly age-appropriate, but there was no getting away from the floppy tone of his trunk muscles. And there was something unusual about his facial features – chin rather small, nose oddly pointed.

'He's due back with the paediatricians soon, isn't he?'

Milly nodded.

'I'll drop them a line, ask them what they think.'

Added together, the various findings were strongly sug-gestive of a genetic syndrome. There are in excess of 5,000 described to date. I'm familiar with the commonest – condi-tions like Downs – but accurate diagnosis of rare and usual cases is very much a specialist pursuit.

The paediatrician agreed something looked amiss so took blood for chromosomal analysis. This picked up an abnormal-ity diagnostic of something called Williams Syndrome. It is rare, affecting around 1 in 18,000 people, so I wasn't surprised I'd never heard of it. I did some book-work. There was some bad news: mild to moderate learning disability, and frequent cardiovascular abnormalities – hence the murmur. But many affected individuals lead full and occupied lives with support. There are intriguing characteristics, too: striking verbal flair and a passion for music. And Williams has been dubbed the 'opposite of autism' – people with the syndrome have extreme-ly sociable and empathic personalities. Sadly, their relatively low IQ coupled with difficulties reading social cues can make relationships problematic, depriving them of the interaction they so thrive on.

Milly brought Ethan back a couple of months on. I was pleased to find her adjusting well to his diagnosis. It had been a huge and life-changing shock, she said, but she and her husband Tim were coming to terms. We had a good conver-sation about how, in earlier eras, individuals with Williams would simply have been accepted by their communities as just that bit different to the norm. And that's how Milly and Tim have decided to approach things: they feel blessed with a son who has his own unique potential and personality, and who will bring as much charm to their family as he may pose challenges.

They've also joined the Williams Syndrome Foundation (WSF), a small charity dedicated to increasing awareness and providing support. Among a whole host of useful information, Milly and Tim have been sent the WSF's 'blue book'. This mirrors the standard 'red book' except that its milestones and charts are adjusted for a typical Williams Syndrome child. So rather than emphasising delay and disability, the blue book stresses the normality of Ethan's development with reference to his Williams Syndrome peers.

The WSF was founded by affected families. It charges a nominal £10 per year for membership, and it must be run largely on volunteer goodwill. The huge difference they make to parents like Milly and Tim, motivated purely by a desire to help others, gave me a renewed optimism for all that is best about our society, and the human heart.

OFF DUTY

SPEECH DAY

I T WAS ONE of those glorious July days. With the sun on the canvas, and the combined respiration of several hundred proud parents and grandparents, the atmosphere inside the speech day marquee was decidedly stuffy. Faces were being fanned with programmes; applauding palms were sweaty. Just as the procession of students collecting trophies and certificates of achievement came to an end, an elderly man in the front row slumped against the woman next to him, then keeled over on to the grass.

It took a short time to extricate myself from where I was sitting. Concerned people were huddled round when I got there. For a moment I thought this might be a full-blown resuscitation drama – he was strikingly grey, and unconscious – but a swift check established that he was breathing and had a pulse. I sent someone to call for an ambulance, but within a couple of minutes he had fully come round. I took a brief history and he denied any symptoms to suggest anything seriously awry. His colour was pinking up nicely. He started to profess embarrassment at creating such a fuss. It looked like nothing more than a simple faint.

This sort of situation makes you realise how naked you are as a doctor without equipment and technology. I had nothing with which to conduct an examination or tests and, in any case, the setting was far from conducive. Speech day had now finished; people were beginning to traipse out of the marquee, casting curious glances at our tableau – old man on ground; doctor crouched in attendance – as they passed. My two children, desperate to get home and start their summer holidays, were making can-we-go-now faces at me. My patient sat himself up, protesting that he now felt fine. I was on the verge of helping him to his feet and wishing him well, when I noticed the wetness darkening his suit trousers.

People are occasionally incontinent when they faint, but it's rare. I felt uneasy. I thought back to the very first impression I'd had of him, how he had looked dead. I told him I thought he ought to lie back down and wait for the ambulance.

We had a minor battle of wills. His granddaughter was the head girl, he told me, this had been a big day for her, he wanted to rejoin her party. And he had the English distaste for making a scene. He almost persuaded me. When someone came to tell me that the ambulance couldn't negotiate the embankment down to the sports field, and did I really think he needed it, my resolve almost faltered again. But by then I'd pushed him hard for more information, and had elicited the grudging admission that, actually, now I came to mention it, there had been a sudden pain in his stomach and his back before he'd passed out.

My suspicion was confirmed when I phoned the hospital the next day. He was in intensive care having survived emergency surgery for a ruptured aortic aneurysm.

The aorta is the body's main artery, running from the heart, down through the chest and abdomen. Its typical diameter is 2 centimetres. Genetic factors, high blood pressure, and smoking, can all weaken the aortic wall, which then distends, forming a dilatation, or aneurysm. Eventually, stretched thin enough, the artery wall ruptures.

Death is rapid with a catastrophic breach. However, in a small minority of patients – as in this case – the initial 'leak' is sealed by clot, though only temporarily. There follows a variable window during which emergency surgery to graft in an artificial artery may save life – though only half of patients who actually make it to hospital survive.

Aortic aneurysms predominantly affect men, and become increasingly common with age. Diagnosed before they leak or burst, surgical repair is much more feasible, with death rates in the order of 3%. Aneurysms are readily detected by a simple and inexpensive ultrasound scan, and there are good data linking diameter with risk of rupture. For several years, enterprising companies have been offering scans on a private basis, and in 2013 the NHS finished rolling out its own screening programme nationwide. All men are invited for a single scan at age 65. With a normal calibre aorta, the rest-of-life risk is negligible. Aneurysms of greater than 5.5cm diameter have a high chance of rupture, so surgical repair is usually offered. Those in the 'grey zone' are more difficult; at a diameter of 4cm the risks of surgery are about equal to those of leaving alone. Repeat surveillance scans are a way of checking for progression.

I kept in touch with the hospital over the following eleven days, at which point sadly my patient died from kidney failure caused by the massive blood loss he'd sustained. He had at least lived long enough to hear his granddaughter deliver her end-of-year speech as head girl, which must have made him proud. I found out later that she was going on to university to study medicine, something I found particularly poignant. By the time she qualifies as a doctor, the NHS screening programme should have helped reduce mortality from ruptured aortic aneurysms, but it came too late for her family. The memory of that school speech day, and the loss of her grandfather, will stay with her throughout her career.

GIFTS

PERHAPS THE MOST unusual gift I've been given by a patient was when I worked part-time in a rural practice in deepest Norfolk while studying for an MA at the University of East Anglia. The patient in question was a long-retired farm labourer whom I helped through a nasty pneumonia. He wasn't well-off, but at some point in life he had mastered the art of knitting string dishcloths, and he presented me with one as a token of his gratitude. It was more hole than string, but I kept it for several years, so touched was I by the gesture.

During that year, I lived in the village where the practice was located, and it didn't take long for people to learn where the new doctor's house was. From time to time I would arrive home to find a carrier bag dangling from the door handle containing half-a-dozen free-range eggs, or a crop of runner beans, or some other anonymous donation of home produce. This was the mid-1990s, but it was a taste of what life must have been like for country doctors a generation or two before.

The General Medical Council has strict rules on accepting gifts from patients. Great care must be taken to avoid any abuse of trust, and the doctor must ensure that presents don't – or aren't perceived to – affect the treatment a patient is given. A few years ago, back in my home turf in the south-west of England, I looked after a somewhat belligerent businessman who had a non-serious but irksome bowel complaint. Frustrated by his ongoing symptoms he came seeking a specialist referral; he also wanted me to get on the phone and sort it out urgently for him. These requests were made while presenting me with a bottle of extremely fine and extremely expensive wine. I thanked him very much but explained I had to refuse the gift, assuring him that I would care for him exactly as I would anyone else with the same problems.

Easily my most ill-advised acceptance of a gift was when a retired Anglican clergyman registered as a patient around five years ago. In the course of our first consultation, I discovered his life-long involvement in academic theological debate, and was interested to learn that since retiring he'd published two books. I should have known better as a writer myself, but evidently I let myself appear just a little too interested. A couple of days later a parcel appeared in my in-tray containing copies of both esoteric, weighty tomes, with a handwritten note saying he looked forward to hearing my thoughts. Our subsequent consultations were attended by ever-increasing awkwardness as, again and again, I failed to make any comment about them. I found them on my shelves just recently – still unread – when decluttering my room. It made me realise that, at some point in the intervening years, he had simply given up and registered elsewhere, perhaps hoping to find a doctor with more time on his hands for extracurricular advancement.

Under the terms of the contract with the NHS, GPs must maintain a register of any gifts worth more than £100. From time to time in my practice we are left bequests, or a deceased patient's family will ask mourners for donations to the surgery rather than buying funeral flowers. We pay these monies into a separate amenity account, and use the funds to enhance patient care.

Christmas, of course, is a traditional time for giving, and

from early December gifts start to come in from patients. There's always a thumping cake from Mrs Fox, which we hoist to the staff room upstairs and by great collective effort manage to whittle down to a few crumbs and stray raisins over the coming weeks. Other presents come in bottles or boxes – booze in the former, biscuits or chocolates in the latter.

My senior partner, Hugh, gets more than the rest of us put together. In part this reflects his length of service: he was one of the two co-founders of the practice, and has been in post nigh-on 30 years, during which time he's helped a heck of a lot of people. He also has a wonderful bedside manner. He is deeply interested in people, and frequently spends more time in the consultation catching up on what they've been doing, how their family is getting on, where the new house is, and what happened to the dog, than he does in talking about their medical problems.

As a consequence, Hugh is pretty much the essence of all that is good in British general practice. I've lost count of the times one of us has been discussing a perplexing patient over coffee, only for Hugh to fill us in on the key bit of information about who they're related to, or what happened to them in the distant past, which suddenly solves the puzzle.

We'd have lost him years ago if we let him eat and drink everything he's given at Christmas. Instead, everyone's presents are stacked in the practice manager's office – in effect, a Santa's grotto – and in the days leading up to the holiday each staff member is invited to take a share. It's recognition that our practice is only as good as the loyal and dedicated people – receptionists, administrators, nurses, cleaners – who make up our wonderful team.

HEIMLICH

I T MAY HAVE been an overly large chunk of steak; or, perhaps, in my haste to rejoin the conversation, I didn't chew sufficiently, and hurried to swallow. Either way, I felt the food lodge in my throat.

Disconcerted, I sipped some water. The lump slid a little further down. I waited, hoping to feel the resumption of a successful swallow, something we accomplish without a moment's thought countless times each day. Instead, there was an inexorable stretching sensation, with associated discomfort, then a sudden urge to cough.

I didn't have much air in my lungs. The couple of water-strewn coughs I managed were otherwise ineffectual. I tried to draw breath, to get more ammo in there. Not a bit of air shifted. My windpipe was completely blocked.

I'd updated my life support training just a couple of months before. Bizarrely, I could hear the instructor's voice: You'll be sitting in a restaurant, another diner will suddenly start spluttering. If they're giving effective coughs, encourage them and monitor. But if they can't cough effectively then you've got to do something, and pretty damn quick.

I couldn't speak, of course, but my mind was screaming: *I'm choking, someone please help me!*

I lurched to my feet. If you're going to choke, there's no better place than a room full of doctors. The restaurant was packed with us, enjoying an evening meal mid-way through a two-day conference. Those sitting closest jumped up. I heard the word, 'Heimlich', and felt someone's hands come from behind, joining together round my upper abdomen.

At the end of exhalation, a couple of litres of air remain in the lungs. Described in 1974 by Henry Heimlich, an American thoracic surgeon, the Heimlich manoeuvre exploits this 'functional residual capacity'. A sharp in-and-up-thrust beneath the ribs compresses the diaphragm, causing a sudden rise in air pressure within the chest. In theory, this should create enough force to expel the offending foreign body.

The hands from behind yanked hard. Nothing happened. With complete airway obstruction, you've probably got around two minutes till consciousness is lost, and death follows a few minutes later. I've sometimes wondered how I will react when I'm told I'm going to die. Now I have an inkling. There was a degree of panic, but far stronger was the thought: what a stupid, pathetic, embarrassing way to go.

Another abdominal thrust, even harder this time, practically lifted me off the floor. And – amazingly – the offending lump of steak flew right out of my mouth. I breathed again, relishing the sensation of air flooding my lungs.

It was over in a blur. People checked I was OK, I thanked my rescuer – Nick, a fellow GP from a nearby city – and we all took our seats again. I doubt Debrett's covers the etiquette of this situation. I felt a ludicrous social obligation to remain at table. A few jokes were cracked, everyone professed themselves amazed, and someone checked both Nick's and my pulse rates to see who was the more adrenaline-pumped (Nick, apparently). I couldn't face eating. After a couple of minutes, another colleague, noting my pallor, gently enquired if I wanted to excuse myself.

Back in my hotel room, the shock hit full force. I kept re-experiencing the sensation of being unable to breathe, and ruminating on what had so nearly happened. I slept poorly. I left in the morning; I had an overwhelming desire to be home.

For GPs, true emergencies occur only rarely, yet we must be able to respond swiftly and automatically when they do. To this end, we update our life support training annually. I've practised the Heimlich manoeuvre on resuscitation dummies many times, and invariably wonder how it would go were I to have to perform it for real. Corresponding with Nick afterwards, I discovered that was the abiding legacy for him: relief, almost disbelief, that his training had proved so spectacularly effective. With 200 UK deaths from choking each year, I'm extremely glad it did.

In 2016, Henry Heimlich was living in a retirement home in Ohio when a female fellow-resident started choking on a piece of steak. Heimlich, then 96, had never before had a chance to put his own technique into practice. He leapt to his feet, performed the famous abdominal thrust, and neatly cleared the blockage that was preventing the woman from breathing. Heimlich died a few months later, and I can't help feeling he went happy in the knowledge that he had joined the ranks of the estimated 40,000 people who have saved a fellow human being's life with the manoeuvre that he devised.

POOL TOE

THE BRUTAL HEAT wave affecting Southern Europe in 2016 became known among locals as 'Lucifer'. Having holidayed in Italy that summer, I fully understood the nickname. An early excursion caused the beginnings of sunstroke in two of our family, so we abandoned plans to explore the cultural heritage of the Amalfi region and strayed no further than five metres from the hotel pool for the rest of the week.

The children were delighted, of course, particularly my twelve-year-old step-daughter, Gracie, who proceeded to spend hours at a time playing in the water. Towelling herself after one long session, she noticed something odd.

'What's happened there?' she asked, holding her foot aloft in front of my face.

I inspected the proffered appendage: on the underside of her big toe was an oblong area of glistening red flesh looking like a chunk of raw steak.

'Did you injure it?'

She shook her head. 'It doesn't hurt at all.'

I shrugged and said she must have grazed it. She was unconvinced, pointing out – entirely reasonably – that she would remember if she'd done that. She has great faith in plasters, though, and once it was dressed she forgot all about it. I dismissed it, too, assuming it was one-of-those-things.

By the end of the following day, the pulp on the underside of every one of her toes looked the same. As the doctor in the family, I felt under some pressure to come up with an explanation. I made up something about burns from the hot paving slabs around the pool. Gracie didn't say as much, but her look suggested a dawning scepticism over my claims to hold a medical degree.

The next day, Gracie and her new-found holiday playmate, Eve, both abruptly terminated a marathon piggy-in-the-middle session in the pool with Eve's dad.

'Our feet are bleeding,' they announced, somewhat incredulously, on getting out of the water. Sure enough, bright red blood was flowing, apparently painlessly, from the bottoms of their respective big toes.

Doctors are used to contending with Google. Often, what patients discover on the internet causes them undue alarm, and our role is to provide context and reassurance. But not infrequently people turn up information that outstrips our own knowledge. On my return from our room with fresh supplies of plasters, my wife looked up from her sun lounger with an air of quiet amusement.

'It's called Pool Toe,' she said, handing across her iPhone.

The page she'd tracked down described the girls' situation exactly. Friction burns, most commonly seen in children, caused by repetitive hopping about on the abrasive floors of swimming pools. Doctors practising in hot countries must see it all the time. I doubt it presents that often to British GPs.

I remained puzzled about the lack of pain: the injuries looked dramatic, but neither Gracie nor Eve was particularly bothered. Here the internet drew a blank, but I suspect it is to do with the 'pruning' of our skin that we're all familiar with after a soak in the bath. This only occurs over the pulps of our fingers and toes. It was once thought to be caused by water diffusing into skin cells, making them swell, but the truth is far more fascinating. The wrinkling is an active process, triggered by immersion, where the blood supply to the pulp regions is switched off, causing the skin there to shrink and pucker, creating the biological equivalent of tyre treads on our fingers and toes. This markedly improves grip – of great evolutionary advantage when grasping slippery fish in a river, or if trying to maintain balance on slick wet rocks.

The flip side of this enhanced grip is much greater friction, leading to abrasion of the skin through repeated microtrauma. And the lack of blood flow causes nerves to shut down, depriving us of the pain that would otherwise alert us to the ongoing tissue damage. An adaptation that helped our ancestors hunt in rivers proves considerably less use on a modern summer holiday. I may not have seen much of the local heritage, but the trip to Italy taught me something new all the same.

FLYING

SOMEWHERE OFF THE north African coast the tannoy crackled out a request: 'Any doctor on board please make themselves known to cabin crew'. Most medics harbour a secret apprehension about such scenarios when flying, and I have to confess I paused for a few seconds. No one else sprang to their feet, though. My post-holiday carefree mood was over.

A plump middle-aged Asian woman was slumped in her seat near the front of the cabin. She was hyperventilating; her eyes were closed and she was making only inconsistent responses. She seemed to be travelling alone; certainly none of the startled people in the vicinity owned up to knowing her. It's difficult to convey quite how impossible it is to examine someone in the middle of a row in economy class. Somehow the cabin crew and I managed to extract her and lie her in the aisle.

I set about checking her over, trying to ignore the passengers craning over their seats to take photos on their phones. Initially I was worried about a blood clot lodging in the lung, but the woman's condition quickly improved, and we found enough English in common for me to start honing down the possibilities. By the time a stewardess came to ask whether the captain should divert to Faro in Portugal, I had a pretty good idea it wouldn't be necessary.

Flying at altitude presents physiological challenges: cabin pressure typically equates to conditions on top of a 6,000 foot mountain (Britain's highest peak, Ben Nevis, is around 4,400 feet). This causes a drop of around 10% in blood oxygen saturation, which healthy people won't notice, but if someone has significant heart or lung disease, or if they're very anaemic, they may run into problems. My patient did indeed appear anaemic. Beyond this, flying can also generate significant psychological stress – being trapped in a speeding metal tube six miles up is deeply unsettling to some, to say nothing of the reasons one might be travelling. My patient was visiting a gravely ill relative. The combination of hypoxic symptoms and underlying anxiety had sent her into full-blown panic.

That ought to have been it: none but the most globe-trotting medic would expect to encounter more than one airborne emergency in their lives. I was relieved that mine had been so benign (perhaps the most famous case occurred in 1995 when orthopaedic professor Angus Wallace, and colleague Tom Wong, had to insert a chest drain to relieve a potentially fatal collapsed lung in a female passenger. They improvised the drain out of a coat hanger and a urinary catheter, sterilising it in Courvoisier cognac before operating.)

I felt jinxed, then, when on another flight a year or so ago the tannoy broadcast the same request. This turned out to be a Londoner in his sixties who'd had nasty gastroenteritis in the days before travelling. He'd felt really poorly at the airport in Morocco, but had been patched up with an anti-sickness injection by a doctor there and allowed to fly in spite of dehydration. We'd already begun our descent when he collapsed, so I got the captain to radio ahead to have an ambulance meet us on landing. This involved the plane taxiing to a special apron well away from the main terminal. The rest of the passengers were disembarked from one end, while I stayed behind to transfer the patient's care to the paramedics.

By the time the ambulance finally drove off, the entire flight crew had disappeared. I was left to find my own way through the deserted maze of night-time Heathrow's air-side corridors. I caught up with my fellow passengers at reclaim – our luggage was having to be recovered manually, which took absolutely ages – and was berated by a man furious that my actions had caused him such delay.

This July I'm heading for Zambia, my first long-haul flight since then. Believe you me, I wish everyone on board a safe and healthy trip.

INSURANCE

E MMA CAME TO see me following a holiday in the States. She was in New York when cystitis struck. She'd had it a couple of times during her undergraduate years so knew what to do. She upped her water intake, went to Walmart for cranberry juice, and when those measures failed she took herself along to the nearest emergency room to get treatment.

That was where any similarity with her UK experiences ceased. Her NHS doctors had managed her previous bouts with a brief chat and a prescription for an antibiotic. Her American physicians appeared a whole lot more concerned. She had a pelvic examination, urine and swab samples sent to the lab, blood tests, and a first dose of antibiotics administered via a drip. They'd wanted to do a scan, too, but had reluctantly agreed to her deferring this till she was back in Britain. Just as well, really. She'd already racked up over $500 in charges. An ultrasound would have comfortably taken her over the $1000 mark.

There seemed to Emma only two possible explanations: either the NHS had woefully under-treated her in the past, or my American colleagues had been wilfully overdoing it in order to maximise their income. The reality lies somewhere in between. UK medical culture takes a low-key, 'common things are common' approach to many illnesses, only investigating in more detail when it becomes clear that it's required (which might be when there's a lack of response to an initial course of treatment). Across the Atlantic, patients tend to be exhaustively worked up at the outset, as though each and every one is going to prove to be that rare case with something much more complex underlying it.

There is an income consideration in this – American doctors are, broadly speaking, paid for their activity, whereas their British counterparts are encouraged to conserve resources. Of equal importance, though, is the medico-legal culture. American society is unforgiving of apparent delay in definitive diagnosis so doctors practise defensively, with the spectre of lawsuits ever-hanging over them. In the UK, it is accepted that diagnosis is often a multi-stage process. This is good for the majority of patients who avoid the considerable harms that can arise from unnecessary invasive investigations. The flip-side, though, is there may be a time lag in picking up significant pathology. This rarely compromises outcomes, but in some tragic instances it does, and that can be very hard for those affected.

Being young and on a tight budget, and given the premiums charged for cover in the States, Emma had travelled uninsured – something she was now regretting at leisure. Had she holidayed in Europe she would have found insurance considerably cheaper. Not only is European medical culture closer to that at home – though I did once have a patient return from Bulgaria clutching three different drugs and a set of CT scans following a simple bout of sinusitis – but British travellers can, at least until Brexit, apply for a European Health Insurance Card (formerly known as the E111) which entitles them to state healthcare if they're taken ill in a participating country.

The EHIC doesn't obviate the need for travel insurance,

though. In the UK the idea of paying to see a doctor is still anathema, but most European countries levy consultation and hospital inpatient charges on their citizens, so state provision often carries significant costs. France and Germany are among the most expensive; Ireland, Portugal, Italy, and Greece are virtually free (which must say something about the origins of the eurozone crisis).

Those holidaying in more exotic locations may be exposed to serious infectious diseases, which can be life-threatening. Rather than the first-world problem of overzealous doctors, healthcare provision may be sparse and very basic in the destination country. Vaccination, pre-travel advice and information, and adequate insurance to cover medical evacuation are important preparations. I'll be in Zambia when this appears in print, hoping none of what I've put in place will prove necessary. If you're travelling this summer, wherever you're going I wish you a happy and healthy trip.

FIRST WORLD PROBLEMS

Although the flights to and from Zambia that summer proved uneventful, and the travel insurance I'd arranged was never needed, the holiday itself turned out to be the most difficult our family has ever known, as this next column describes.

'**D**AD'S REALLY NOT well,' my wife said, voice so low only I could hear.

There were fourteen of us having lunch on the verandah. My father-in-law was at the end of the table. He'd been under-par for days, but now appeared completely withdrawn. His breathing rate was up. From time to time his arms twitched involuntarily in his lap.

We convened a family con-flab away from the main gathering, and decided to seek medical attention. This being Zambia, there are no GPs – it meant a long drive to one of the hospitals in the nearby, sprawling, Copperbelt town.

Debate ensued as to which. The state facility was dismissed – there'd be no drugs, and few if any staff. The modest numbers of Zambian-trained doctors tend to gravitate to the capital or emigrate after completing their year of compulsory rural service. The oldest local private clinic – which my father-in-law had run for ten years prior to his retirement – had also struggled with recruitment lately. We settled on the Forward – a rival hospital opened earlier in the year, whose Uzbekistani doctors were gaining a good reputation.

My father-in-law was deteriorating. There is no ambulance service; we manhandled him into the 4x4. The rural dirt roads are as red and cratered as a Martian landscape. My wife and I hung on to him as we were thrown about inside the vehicle; he was too weak to keep himself upright. Things were easier once we reached the tarmac of town, but by then he was semi-conscious.

At the Forward, the duty doctor whisked him to the emergency room. My mother-in-law was waylaid by a receptionist seeking a hefty cash deposit. To a Briton, 'private hospital' conjures up spotless environments, attentive nursing staff, expert consultants. In Zambia, it simply means a fighting chance. The clinic possessed one pulse oximeter – a standard bit of kit to monitor blood oxygen – which was held together with tape. The floor was filthy with debris and discarded gloves. Needles and syringes were cast casually into ordinary bins along with the other clinical waste.

Notwithstanding the squalor, the doctors had basic investigations in-house. A chest x-ray and echocardiogram showed fulminant pneumonia and heart failure, and blood tests revealed the resultant clotting and kidney abnormalities that were leading to his precipitous decline. Oxygen and intravenous drugs, including two potent antibiotics I was amazed to find available, produced some temporary improvement. A private ambulance chartered from a South African company took him to visit two other hospitals before a working CT scanner could be found.

Over the coming days we met all five Forward hospital doctors, who did their utmost medically. They had no influence on the nursing staff, however, who remained cloistered in their office, emerging only to administer drugs. The call button didn't work. It was left to family to encourage drink and food, to lift and turn to prevent pressure sores, to toilet, and to raise the alarm on the numerous occasions when the oxygen stopped flowing.

After three days, my father-in-law suffered a stroke and died peacefully, his wife and daughter at his bedside. His health had been declining for several years. He'd known he would have received better care had he returned to the UK, but his love for Africa and her wildlife had been too strong to abandon his adoptive home.

During his final illness, I got various medical social media updates from the UK. The wife of the then Justice Secretary, Michael Gove, was, I learned, disgusted that her husband couldn't get his sore foot x-rayed at a Somerset minor injuries unit on a Sunday afternoon. Hundreds of thousands of people were signing a 'no confidence' petition following Health Secretary Jeremy Hunt's inflammatory and plain-wrong insinuation that the NHS shuts down at weekends.

I want our health service to be as good as it can be, but the juxtaposition with what I was witnessing in Zambia felt raw. UK medical students undertake electives abroad to gain valuable perspectives on healthcare elsewhere in the world. Perhaps it's time our politicians did likewise.

IN HOURS

NOT SEEING FOR LOOKING

EDNA PHONED; SHE thought she had a urine infection. Older women are particularly prone: the lack of oestrogen after the menopause leads to thinning of the vulval tissues, allowing bacteria easier entry to the bladder. Additionally, reduced mobility and social contact mean the elderly often don't drink enough, so germs tend not to get 'flushed out', and more readily take hold.

Symptoms aren't always typical. Whereas younger woman experience pain passing water, and need to make frequent, urgent trips to the loo, very often older patients simply become confused and go 'off legs'. That said, Edna's symptoms did sound characteristic: she was peeing every hour, and she couldn't hang on too long when she had to go.

I called on her during the lunchtime round. Home visits take up a lot of time, but they are a vital service for the housebound. Like most doctors, I find them enlightening – nothing beats seeing someone in their own environment for getting a handle on their bigger picture. Edna's house was clean and tidy, she was neatly dressed and was steady on her feet when she came to the door – all signs that, whatever was wrong with her, she was managing to keep things on track.

She'd collected a specimen, so after a brief chat I disappeared to her bathroom to test it. This involves dunking a reagent strip into the sample. These 'dipsticks' have ten different test pads in a row, each of which undergoes colour change if they encounter a specific chemical. There are several that might indicate infection – blood, protein, infection-fighting cells, and bacterial breakdown products called nitrites. Edna's sample was negative for all four.

I returned to her sitting room and questioned her more closely. In typical cystitis, the bladder feels full-to-bursting but the actual volumes passed are surprisingly small. Edna was quite clear she was peeing buckets. This could have been a symptom of diabetes mellitus – excess sugar filters out through the kidneys, dragging large volumes of water along with it – but Edna's dipstick had been negative for glucose, too, ruling that out.

There's a different form of diabetes – diabetes insipidus – which has nothing to do with sugar levels. In DI, a hormone system that regulates water balance goes awry, causing the kidneys to continue pumping out urine even though the body is dehydrating. It's rare, but can be associated with serious underlying conditions.

I came across to where Edna was sitting and examined her carefully, but there was nothing to suggest dehydration. The only other thing I could think of was heart failure. Fluid accumulates in the legs under the influence of gravity, causing them to become markedly swollen. When they're elevated, the water floods back into the circulation, producing a surge in urine output. That tends to occur at night, though, when the person lies flat. In any case, Edna didn't have many signs of heart failure, either.

I was stumped. Crouched beside her chair, I launched into a wordy explanation of what I thought we should do next, which basically involved a lot of tests. She listened politely, but I could tell she wasn't interested. She just wanted me to solve the problem. Her loo is upstairs, and she was worn out with traipsing up and down all the time.

It was then that I saw it: a pint glass on the occasional table beside her, half full of water. I asked about it. Oh yes, she said, that's my daughter, she's been on at me for not drinking enough – says it's a sure-fire way to get a urine infection. I asked how much she was drinking. Pints and pints of the stuff, she told me, had been all week, ever since her daughter had visited.

I'd been so busy looking for medical causes that I'd missed the blindingly obvious. Edna was tipping gallons in the top end, only for it to reappear again in the time-honoured fashion. Feeling foolish – though also amused that she hadn't made the connection herself – I suggested a more measured approach to maintaining fluid intake. Her symptoms settled within a day.

CATCHER

To BEGIN WITH, it seemed Barry's wrists were the problem. He told me about the pain he was experiencing, the pins and needles that came and went in his hands. I started to examine him. His palms were calloused, fingers thick and stubby, veterans of the heavy work he'd undertaken throughout his fifty-seven years. Even as I assessed this first problem, he mentioned his knees. I moved on to look at those. Then it was his back. I couldn't get to grips with one thing before he veered to the next.

I teach my registrars to be aware how a consultation is making them feel: that can give valuable clues as to the patient's own emotional state. Barry was making me feel overwhelmed – the more so as I learned that he'd been experiencing all these problems for years.

'Why are you coming about them now,' I asked, 'rather than six months ago, or in six months' time?'

'I need some time off, doc.'

There was something about the way he wouldn't meet my gaze. And that feeling of being overwhelmed.

'What's going on at work?'

His tone hardened as he told me how he'd lost it a couple of days before. How one of the others had been winding him up, and something inside him had snapped, and he'd taken a swing at his workmate and landed a punch. Barry had walked out and hadn't been back since. I tried to find out if he'd heard from his boss about it; if he knew what was likely to happen next. He told me he didn't care.

We talked some more. I learned that he'd been uncharacteristically short-tempered for months; his partner was fed up with being shouted at. Sleep had gone to pot, and Barry had taken to drinking heavily to knock himself out at night. He was smoking twice his usual amount. Men like Barry often don't experience depression as classic low mood and tearfulness; they get rage-filled and turn in on themselves, repelling those closest to them in the process.

Depression is a complex condition, with roots that can frequently be traced right back to childhood experiences, but bouts tend to be precipitated by problems with relationships, work, money, or health. In Barry's case, the main factor turned out to be his job. He had been an HGV driver, but at the start of the year his company had lost its operator's licence. To keep the business afloat, his boss had diversified. Barry hated what he now had to do. Barry was now a catcher.

I didn't know what that meant. Getting up at the crack of dawn, he told me, driving to some factory farm somewhere, entering huge sheds and spending hours catching chickens, thousand upon thousand of them, shoving them into crates, stashing the crates on to a lorry, working under relentless pressure to get the sheds cleared and the birds off to the next stage of the food production chain.

'It's a young man's game,' he told me. 'It's crippling me, all that bending and catching.'

It wasn't really his joints, though. Men like Barry can find it hard to talk about difficult emotion, but it was there in his eyes. I had a sudden understanding: Barry, capturing bird after panicking bird, stuffing them into the transport containers, the air full of alarmed clucking and dislodged feathers. Hour after hour of it. It was traumatising him, but he couldn't admit anything so poncey.

'I just want to get back to driving.'

That would mean landing a new job, and he doubted he would be able to do so, not at his age. And he couldn't take just any old work: he had to earn a decent enough wage to keep up with a still sizeable mortgage. His sense of hopelessness was palpable. We talked about how antidepressants might improve his symptoms, and made a plan to tackle the alcohol. I signed him off to give him some respite, and the chance to look for new work – the one thing that was going to resolve his depression. Currently, he felt as trapped as the chickens he found himself cornering day after soul-destroying day.

Barry didn't return when his sick note ran out, and it was over a year before I saw him again. At the end of the consultation about a minor, unrelated matter, he thanked me for what I had done, told me he had found himself a new job back driving lorries, and felt as happy and healthy as he had always done.

REUNION

GORDON WAS PROBABLY the sickest patient ever to walk into my practice. He turned up at the front desk one morning asking, between snatched breathes, to book an appointment sometime in the next week or so, when convenient. A good GP receptionist is worth any amount of gold. Gaby took one look at him, instructed him to take a seat, then rang to tell me I needed to fit him in straight after my current patient.

He was in crashing left-ventricular failure, his heart muscle no longer pumping blood effectively, his skin pale and clammy, and his lungs as sodden as wet sponges. He'd had some chest pain several days previously, which he hadn't wanted to make a fuss about, and sure enough it had settled after a few hours. That would have been the massive heart attack that had killed off much of his heart muscle. His breathing had been getting progressively more laboured ever since until, in the end, he'd thrown in the towel and decided he ought to see someone.

I gave him immediate intravenous treatment then sent him in by 999 ambulance. He survived a cardiac arrest in hospital, was an inpatient for another week or so, and came out on a panoply of medications already looking and feeling distinctly better.

He was accompanied by one or other of his grown-up daughters to his first few follow-up appointments. The experience had shocked them and they weren't about to let their father's taciturn stoicism get in the way of him seeking proper care again. They were also determined to get him to clean up his act: no more cigarettes, and the whisky would have to go as well. But as we tinkered with his tablets over the coming months, and as Gordon grew ever stronger, the shockwaves from the crisis gradually dissipated. Both daughters had young families and busy lives of their own. Gordon started to attend surgery on his own.

It was then that I learned about his hinterland. How he'd lost his beloved wife Maggie, who had been his childhood sweetheart, to cancer the year before. With both his children settled in south-west England it had made sense to move, so he'd packed up and left Scotland behind. It was good to be near his kids, he told me, and he liked being a grandad well enough. Although what he said sounded superficially optimistic, his tone was weary, as though the words weighed a great deal and took a lot of effort to drag out. I got a strong sense of how it must be, returning to his flat after each visit to his daughters' happy families, back to his memories of Maggie and the unfamiliar place that was now home.

Depression is a normal part of grieving, but if it takes a firm hold then it can sap us of the motivation and energy to adapt to life changes. He agreed to start treatment, and after a while he seemed to respond. He got back in touch with old friends from school and workdays, and had a couple of trips away with them.

But when he talked about these renewed connections, there was always wistfulness in his voice. He didn't need to explain: everything was a pale substitute for the retirement he and Maggie had looked forward to together. Whisky crept back in, first as a few drams when he met up with old friends, latterly as a resumption of his habitual late-night consolation. And booze wasn't the same without a fag in hand. He wanted his pleasures back, he explained; life was about more than simply keeping on.

He thanked me for what I'd done, but said he wouldn't need to see me again. A few months later, one of his daughters rang to say he'd been found dead in his flat – another heart attack. I wondered if it had taken him swiftly, or whether he'd felt the familiar pain and welcomed it – resolved, this time, not to make any more calls that might delay his reunion with Maggie.

FEAR

DAVID DIDN'T WAIT to sit down. 'I want you to check my kidney.'

His tone was aggressive, command rather than request. He laid a hand on his back, much lower than where patients typically experience renal pain.

'And I've got to tell you,' he said, 'I wasn't impressed with your colleague at all. I saw her a couple of months ago about my breathing – she had a thoroughly unprofessional manner. I want your opinion on my lungs as well.'

I glanced at his notes while he took a seat. His last consultation had been six months previously, when he'd expected four different issues to be dealt with in the space of ten minutes. Emma had tackled indigestion, knee pain, a lump on the arm, and had somehow managed to squeeze in a comprehensive respiratory examination at the end. She would have been incredibly brisk and focused. Or, as David clearly saw it, unprofessional.

'Which did you want to address today?' I asked.

'Sorry?'

'The kidney or the breathing? We'll start with the one that's most pressing, and if we run out of time then we'll book another appointment.'

David gave an incredulous snort. 'I'd have thought, as a *doctor*, you'd be more interested in my health than your time.'

He'd really irritated me by now – rude, inconsiderate,

demanding. But unless a patient is actually being abusive, professional ethics require us to overcome personal feelings and keep our focus on good care.

'I very much want to look after your health,' I assured him, trying a smile. 'I just want to make sure we have the time to do so properly.'

That seemed to mollify him a little. He decided his kidney was the priority, and that the breathing issues – unchanged for the past six months – could wait if needed. I took a brief history of the pain in his back, present for the past few weeks, then sent him to the loo to produce a sample.

His urine tested clear. Abdominal examination was hampered by obesity, but I found nothing untoward in the kidney region. I stood him up and checked his back, pointing out how tight it was when he stretched down to his left, and how tender the lumbar muscles were on the other side.

I explained all the reasons I thought his symptoms were due to a back strain, and nothing to do with his kidney at all. Given how fixed he'd seemed on the idea of a renal cause, and how prickly his manner had been, I was expecting a battle. But he readily accepted my verdict and started to gather his things. I asked if he wanted to talk about his shortness of breath now.

'No, no, it's fine. Your colleague put it down to my weight.' He patted his stomach. 'I expect she's right.'

The change in his manner was remarkable. He paused with his hand on the door. 'I'm a friend of Tom Blackstone's,' he told me. 'I thought the same thing was happening to me.'

'Ah,' I said. 'I see.'

As I typed up my notes, everything slotted into place. Tom had presented with abdominal pain last year, and it had turned out to be due to a renal tumour. Unfortunately, the cancer had already spread to his chest by the time it was diagnosed. When David had developed pain where he believed his kidney to be, it had alarmed him. And suddenly, the getting out of puff when climbing stairs – attributed to weight six months previously – must have struck him in a newly sinister light.

Fear and anger are very close cousins. As David had become convinced that he, too, must have metastatic kidney cancer, he would have reinterpreted Emma's earlier hurried assessment as a negligent missed opportunity. He'd come armed for war, determined to make damn sure the next doctor wasn't going to let him down the same way.

A few patients are habitually unpleasant, but most of the aggression and frustration we sometimes encounter reflects how frightened and vulnerable any of us can feel when our health looks suddenly to be on the line.

COLIN AND MARY

A N ADVERT ON a bus shelter caught my eye recently. The gist was: If you're over sixty and you feel the slightest bit peaky, you'd best get yourself along to the doctor, because illness can be so much more serious at that kind of age. It filled me with gloom. There seems no room for common sense any more; everything must be devolved to a professional. The logic – encourage people to seek help at the first hint of trouble and you'll catch anything major at an early stage – is seductive yet flawed. Waves of worried-well suck vast amounts of time out of the health service, to the detriment of those with important disease. Even important diseases can be vague and undifferentiated in their initial phases, making them hard to diagnose. And then there's the psychological downside of continually sapping people's confidence in their own judgement.

Having said that, the folk who devise these awareness-raising campaigns mean well, and there is certainly another side to the coin. The advert put me in mind of Colin and Mary. They were an unusual couple, she in her late seventies, he some fifteen years her junior, and they were devoted to each other. They'd never had children, and kept themselves to themselves, rarely bothering with doctors – in part, perhaps, because Colin was tired of being nagged about his inveterate smoking. It was highly unusual to be asked to visit Mary.

She was sitting in their somewhat dingy lounge when I

arrived. And that was the problem, Colin explained: Mary had been 'right as rain' the previous day, but now he couldn't get her off the sofa. I asked her various questions, but she denied pain or any other symptoms. She just couldn't move.

Although not typical, I wondered about a stroke – her speech was halting and unclear, and her limbs were markedly stiff – but she firmly declined hospital admission. I set about getting some urgent home care for them, and sent off a battery of investigations to try to get to the bottom of it.

Ultimately, the only condition that seemed to explain Mary's presentation was Parkinson's disease, in which the area of the brain – the substantia nigra – responsible for executing voluntary movements slowly degenerates. The problem was, Parkinson's takes years to develop, and Mary had succumbed overnight. The only time I'd come across such an acute onset was when a drug had caused Parkinson's-like side-effects, but Mary hadn't been prescribed anything new for ages.

I cross-examined Colin in detail. It turned out his 'right as rain' had been hideously misleading. Mary had been becoming progressively less mobile for a long time, which they'd been putting down to old age. In the weeks prior to her final seizing-up, Colin had been having literally to manhandle her across the room. Trying to get her upstairs had involved putting her over his shoulder and shoving with Herculean determination. It was an eye-wateringly scary picture.

Mary soon improved with treatment – there are a number of drugs that supplement the neurotransmitter dopamine that becomes depleted with the degeneration of the substantia nigra. The whole episode raised an altogether more delicate issue: what to do when a patient or their carer seems to lack the kind of common sense that would see most people seeking professional help? We had carefully to evaluate Mary's competence to make decisions about her care, and the degree to which Colin's disregard for the medical profession might be exerting an undue influence. In the end, we had to move her to a nursing home.

Some months later, Colin succumbed at home to a smoking-related cancer, declining all but the minimum of help right to the end. His was an almost pathological stoicism, and I can imagine the disdain he would have felt for that bus shelter advert. That was his right, of course, but the tragedy was that, in the end, Mary had needed protection from his very particular brand of loving care.

HEALTH CHECK

Fifty-year-old Graham was an infrequent attender, and his only recent consultation was a couple of months previously, when he'd come for his NHS Health Check. I saw from the notes that my nursing colleague had found a borderline risk of heart disease – a bit overweight, blood pressure a little up – so I prepared myself for a discussion about the issues.

But it wasn't that at all. I noticed Graham limping as he walked to my consulting room.

'I thought it was just a sprain,' he told me, slipping his shoe and sock off. 'But it won't settle down.'

I quizzed him about the history. Yes, he'd turned the ankle. Yes, it went on to swell over the outer side. He'd done all the right things – ice, rest, compression bandaging – but although the swelling had improved, he was still getting pain a couple of months later, and his foot felt distinctly unstable.

The ankle is far and away the commonest sprain site we see. All joints are kept within their usual range of motion by a combination of bone anatomy and fibrous ligaments. Put enough force in the wrong direction, though, and the joint can be made to move in ways nature never intended. The ligaments stretch and tear, causing the familiar pain and swelling. But usually things repair themselves with time and rest.

Examining Graham's foot, though, I noticed something very odd. We're all familiar with the bony lumps at either side of our ankles – the medial and lateral malleoli, to give them their proper names. Sliding about in front of Graham's lateral malleolus were a couple of rope-like structures that ought not to have been there. Though I've seen countless ankle injuries over the years, it was the first time I'd encountered this particular variety.

'You've subluxed your peroneal tendons,' I told him, much to his bemusement.

The movements of our feet and ankles are controlled by the muscles in our lower legs. The peroneal muscles lie at the outside of the calf, and form two tendons that hook round the back of the lateral malleolus before running forward to attach to the bones of the foot. They're held behind the lateral malleolus by an extremely tough ligament called the retinaculum. Tear that, and there's nothing to stop them popping out of place, rendering the peroneal muscles effectively useless.

The most famous sufferer of this injury was Gareth Bale, the Welsh star striker, who tore his right retinaculum during his club, Real Madrid's, successful 2016 Champions' League campaign. Bale ended up having his fixed by top surgeons at a private hospital in London.

While surgery is usually necessary once the injury is established, if diagnosed early enough it is possible to effect a reasonable result (though not good enough for a top-class athlete) by immobilising the ankle in a plaster cast and allowing the retinaculum to heal without interference from the wayward tendons.

'When did you say you did it?' I asked, wondering if Graham might still be suitable for casting.

He looked a bit sheepish. 'The day I came for my health check,' he said. He'd been shocked to hear about his heart disease risk. As soon as he'd got home, he'd looked out his old tracksuit and dusted off an ancient pair of trainers, then set off at a canter round the field behind his house. He'd intended to turn his life around. All he'd ended up turning was his ankle.

NHS Health Checks, offered at five-yearly intervals between the ages of 40-74, have been widely criticised as a waste of money. The idea seems sound: an opportunity to pick up people at risk and help them avoid future health problems. But the theory doesn't match reality: no study has yet found any concrete improvements in actual disease outcomes for the £450 million spent annually on the programme. And while it's assumed that the advice dished out can only have a benign, positive impact, in Graham's case at least, his overly enthusiastic response has left him distinctly worse off, and will end up costing the NHS a few thousand for an operative repair.

MUSINGS

A SENSE OF THE HUMOURS

OUR CULTURE TODAY bears the imprint of a long-passed system of medicine. From the time of Hippocrates in Ancient Greece through to the dawn of scientific medicine in the nineteenth century, human temperament was understood in terms of four humours that were thought to exist within the body – blood, phlegm, yellow bile and black bile. Imbalances between these humours were responsible for different moods and character traits – sanguine, phlegmatic, choleric and melancholic are all terms still in use today. Good health was felt to reflect a state in which the four humours were in balance; diseases arose when they were not.

Each humour was ascribed qualities blended from four natural states – hot, cold, dry and wet. Blood, for example, was hot and wet; phlegm, wet and cold. Dependent on which humour was thought to be in surfeit or deficit, doctors would recommend changes in diet, environment and lifestyle directed towards restoring balance. Physicians' enthusiasm for therapeutic procedures such as blood-letting and purging also arose from the same concerns.

Some of the concepts are remarkably enduring. Despite knowing about viruses, we still talk of having caught a 'cold'. Draughts, or being rain-soaked in a chill wind, are frequently blamed, and we believe that wrapping up and staying warm is essential for recovery – to say nothing of the restorative powers of hot chicken soup. Equally, when someone's burning up with a fever, we may reach for the paracetamol, but we're just as likely to try to cool their blood with a damp flannel applied to the forehead. And the idea that you should starve a fever and feed a cold has continued currency.

Some of the practices of humoral medicine were highly damaging. Draining someone of blood is rarely a good idea (though, interestingly, we still bleed patients with diseases involving iron overload or excess red blood cell production). Other ideas, while misguided, were more benign. Different foodstuffs were ascribed hot, cold, dry and wet properties, and would be advised as remedies for various conditions, either ingested or applied as poultices. Many new mothers today suffering from mastitis will still be told to place a cabbage leaf on the inflamed breast.

While humoral medicine lacked truly effective treatments, it did possess a wisdom that became drowned out by the heady advances of the scientific era. Exercise regimes were a frequent component of a humoral doctor's prescription. Today we are re-emphasising the value of physical activity in a wide range of conditions from depression and stress through to heart disease and type 2 diabetes. A change of environment and partaking of 'fresh air' were frequently prescribed, something modern-day researchers into the health-effects of pollution, or the sense of wellbeing that connection with nature and green space can bring, would readily recognise. And as for diet, the need for balance and moderation is an ongoing concern.

Relaxation and sleep would have been key considerations for a humoral physician. The award of the Nobel Prize in Medicine 2017 to three American scientists for uncovering the workings our internal body clock has thrown new light on how modern lifestyles clash with biology to the detriment of our health. Fully fifty percent of us now routinely get less than six hours sleep - blunting our cognitive abilities, impairing our immunity, and playing havoc with our metabolism. A humoral doctor would have instantly recognised the problem, and would have had a great deal to say about it.

If someone is in poor health then there are likely to be myriad contributors. Some, like genes or age, we can do little about. But what we eat, how much rest and recreation we grant ourselves, what exercise we take, our sense of security and autonomy, and our levels of deprivation, are all important determinants that can be addressed - some at a personal level, others socio-politically. The success of scientific medicine has lead to the belief that there's a pill to solve every ill. Our medical forebears would be astounded by the efficacy of our drugs, but equally bemused by our inability to take care of ourselves.

ANTIBIOTICS

S HORTLY AFTER I joined my practice, my senior
partner gave me a memoir to read. It was written by a
doctor, Kenneth Lane, who had worked in the area from the
late 1920s. As I read stories from his forty-year career, I was
struck by Lane's detailed knowledge of the natural course of
infectious diseases, something entirely unfamiliar to my generation. In the case of a child with pneumonia, for example,
Lane would prepare the parents for each deterioration they
could expect over the first 8-10 days, culminating in the 'pneu-
monic crisis' – a crescendo in fever, hypoxia and delirium
– that would, in a quarter of cases, prove fatal. Only once the
crisis had been survived would Lane start to talk about the
possibility of recovery.

Lane never lost the awe he experienced when, in the late
1940s, the first antibiotics became available. Suddenly, feared
diseases like diphtheria, pneumonia, and scarlet fever could
be cured within a matter of days. To a doctor used to watching impotently as otherwise fit young people died, these new
drugs were miraculous.

I wonder what he would make of the way we use them
today. Around 35 million prescriptions for antibiotics are
issued each year in the UK, the majority for respiratory infections (coughs, colds, sore throats, sinusitis, earache). Studies
have repeatedly shown that in these scenarios antibiotics
do little or no good. The infections are going to get better

anyway, and antibiotics don't reduce serious complications, which are, in any event, rare. They do shorten symptom-duration by about half-a-day on average but, in return, up to 10% of patients experience side effects. And there is now good evidence that antibiotic use interrupts the development of a robust immune response, meaning individuals are susceptible to contracting further infections in the future. The more you use antibiotics, the more you are going to end up using them.

This dismal situation wastes the NHS tens of millions of pounds a year, but the money is trivial compared with the problem of resistance. Bacteria multiply extraordinarily quickly and in huge numbers. This vast-scale, rapid reproduction ensures that, if exposed to an antibiotic, a gene mutation will soon arise that protects the bacterium from the drug's mode of action. The resultant 'resistant' organism will survive and reproduce, its progeny quickly replacing the susceptible strain that is dying all around it. The more antibiotics there are swilling around in the community, the more stimulus there is for resistance to arise. To compound matters, genes for resistance are readily transmitted by a process known as plasmid exchange: once one bacteria has figured out how to evade a particular antibiotic, the capacity spreads like wildfire.

Over the past thirty years, treatment failure – where an infectious bacteria is no longer sensitive to the antibiotic prescribed – has gone from being an occasional phenomenon to something encountered routinely. Some first-line antibiotics have fallen into disuse because they can no longer be relied upon. And it's becoming ever more common for bacteria to be multi-drug resistant, so second- and even third-line antibiotics also fail to kill them. In these cases, and if the infection is serious or life-threatening, there remain 'last line' drugs – agents whose use is permitted only when eradicating otherwise incurable organisms.

Despite this strict control over their use, resistance to these 'last line' antibiotics started to appear around 2007 (probably imported from abroad) and is growing exponentially. We are facing the very real prospect of routinely encountering infectious diseases that we simply cannot treat – a situation that doctors like Kenneth Lane were depressingly familiar with in the pre-antibiotic era. The threat is so alarming that in September 2013 the Department of Health (DoH) launched a strategy to try to tackle the problem.

One approach is to incentivise the pharmaceutical industry to develop new agents. Over the past 15 years only a handful of novel antibiotics have been launched, and at the moment there are virtually none in trials phase. Antibiotic courses are short, and any new agents tend to be reserved for 'last line' use. The resultant small-volume sales make research and development economically unviable under the current drugs patent regime. A different model is needed.

Important as novel drugs will be, the core of the DoH's strategy is to promote responsible 'stewardship' of our existing antibiotics. Surgeries and pharmacies are currently festooned with posters advising against antibiotic use. Not all patients habitually consult doctors with self-limiting infections, but those who do frequently believe antibiotics are essential, and can be doggedly persistent in their efforts to obtain them. Their beliefs usually have their roots in years of inappropriate prescribing. The reasons why doctors prescribe unnecessarily are complex: desire to appear to be helpful; aversion to conflict; blanket treatment 'just in case' serious infection is brewing; ignorance; and time and workload pressures meaning a prescription is used as a quick way to end a consultation.

We need to emphasise the skills that would have been second-nature to someone like Kenneth Lane. His long experience observing infectious diseases enabled him readily to identify potentially serious cases among the morass of self-limiting infections. If he wasn't sure, he would review the patient repeatedly until the diagnosis was clear. We also need to recover the respect Lane had for the antibiotic wonderdrugs that revolutionised his practice. He would, I am sure, be aghast at the casual complacency with which we have come to employ them, and the mess we've got ourselves into as a result.

TOO MUCH MEDICINE

SOMETHING PECULIAR IS going on in the United States – thyroid cancer rates are soaring. It is 300% more prevalent than it was 30 years ago, making it the fastest increasing malignancy in America. Treatment is by removal of the gland. The operation is difficult. The thyroid sits in the neck, just in front of the windpipe, and inadvertent damage to important structures, including the nerves that control the vocal cords, is not uncommon.

Still, if you've got cancer, and a delicate operation is required to cure it, then an operation is what you're going to want, no matter the risks. And you won't mind lifelong treatment with thyroid hormone replacement afterwards, either.

Thankful survivors have joined a campaign, 'Light of Life', to raise awareness of the disease. A 'purple scarf' motif has become their banner, in much the same way that UK breast cancer charities have adopted the 'pink ribbon'. Adverts urge people to 'check your neck', or, more precisely, to ask a doctor to check it for you.

Yet over the same 30-year period, death rates from thyroid cancer have remained resolutely unchanged: no more Americans will die from the disease this year than succumbed to it in 1983. One possible explanation is that US doctors are getting better at treating it, saving ever more lives among the escalating numbers of affected individuals. That would be good if it were true, but the reality is very different: the burgeoning incidence of 'thyroid cancer' is actually an artefact of medical technology, and patients are being subjected to unnecessary treatment.

To understand this, you need to know about VOMIT – victims of medical imaging technology. The acronym was coined in 2003 by Richard Hayward, a consultant neuro-surgeon at Great Ormond Street Hospital. The more suc-cessful we become at imaging the body, the more abnor-malities we find that we don't know how to interpret. Take a random sample of healthy *New Statesman* readers and put them through a CT scanner, for example, and around 25% would prove to have an unsuspected lump in an organ somewhere.

American doctors, with ready access to expensive tech-nologies, and a morbid fear of litigation should they 'miss' something, rely heavily on imaging. Chest CT, routinely used to assess lung symptoms, takes in the thyroid gland, as do MRI scans performed to investigate neck pain. Around 16% of these scans turn up incidental lumps in the thyroid, most of which are too small even to feel on examination.

Having raised an alarm, something more invasive – a biopsy – follows. Tissue from the thyroid lump is examined under the microscope by a pathologist, and that's where the problem is compounded. Pathologists are good at recognising thyroid cancer – they've spent their careers analysing samples obtained from aggressive tumours that have presented clini-cally as enlarging masses. And the tissue from these inciden-tal lumps is often indistinguishable from clinically important cancers, setting in train the full curative machine. But most of the operations are unnecessary. A Japanese study, pub-lished in 2010, followed 340 such patients who volunteered for surveillance rather than surgery. Only a tiny minority had any tumour growth, and some lumps actually regressed during the six years of follow-up. No one came to any harm.

Cancer, long the feared foe, is evidently a more nuanced beast than we have appreciated. For every tumour capable of causing disease or death, many more lie dormant – or are dealt with by our immune systems – and never progress. Powerful imaging technologies developed in recent decades mean we can now detect these indolent cancers, but we have no way of predicting which can be safely left alone.

The problem is not unique to the thyroid gland, nor to the US. It's now accepted that for every life saved by the UK national breast screening programme, another 3 women are diagnosed and aggressively treated for a screen-detected cancer that would never have actually caused disease. And each year thousands of men are diagnosed with prostate cancer that won't ever pose them a problem.

It's a horrible dilemma for patients caught up in the process: cancer provokes inevitable fear. Even given the option of surveillance, most people will choose radical treatment, with all the attendant side-effects and risks. Better safe than sorry. Until we can reliably predict the behaviour of the 'cancers' we are detecting by screening or by accident, doctors are, arguably, causing as much – or even more – harm than good.

Overdiagnosis of cancer is one of the conundrums that has inspired the 'Too Much Medicine' campaign, an international medical movement concerned with the damage modern medicine is capable of inflicting, albeit with the best of intentions. It is in its infancy but has already inspired a series of conferences, and numerous articles in the world's top medical journals. The notion that we can be harmed by having too much medicine looks set to become an increasingly important consideration in the coming years.

CONSENT

I T IS STRAIGHTFORWARD to provide medical care to a child of, say, four. You seek consent from a parent, usually they grant it, then you roll up your sleeves and do the necessary, insulating yourself as best you can from any howls of protest from the actual patient. Fast-forward ten years, though, to when life's journey has brought your patient to the foothills of adulthood, and things are more complex.

It was only in 1986 that the right of a child under 16 to consent to medical treatment was legally established. A mother of five girls, Victoria Gillick, sought to prohibit doctors from providing contraception without her knowledge to any of her daughters whilst they were under 16. The case went all the way to the House of Lords where a judgement delivered by Lord Fraser ruled that, providing a child had sufficient understanding and maturity, they could consent to medical treatment irrespective of their age. It has since become commonplace for doctors to gauge this understanding and maturity – the so-called 'Fraser competence' of a minor – and, where competence is established, to involve them in decisions about their care. And whilst doctors are expected to encourage parental involvement, the prime importance of confidentiality means it need not be insisted upon if the child does not wish their parents to be informed.

Parents cannot overrule consent given by a Fraser-competent child. Paradoxically, if a competent minor

withholds consent for care that is felt to be in their best in-
terests, a parent or a court can override their decision. Such
cases are rare – usually time and careful discussion will effect
resolution – but they do illustrate an important point: we're
prepared to grant autonomy where our children agree with the
prevailing orthodoxy, but we're reluctant to allow them the
freedom to make perverse decisions. This must have its roots
in an appreciation that medical procedures are often scary
and, no matter how competent our children appear to be, we
suspect they're still too influenced by fear to be allowed an
absolutely free rein.

No such protection applies beyond 18: once we reach adulthood, we can decide whatever we like, even if refusing consent
to treatment means we will die. Perhaps the most difficult
challenge, though, comes when dealing with patients aged 16
and 17. These adolescents are legally presumed, by virtue of
their age, to have capacity to consent – there's no requirement
to assess Fraser competence. Yet unlike over-18s they can still,
in theory, have a refusal to consent overridden by someone
with parental authority or by a court. This 16-17 age-band can
pose the most acute of dilemmas, as a tragic case in my area
illustrated all too starkly.

The patient was a youth called Ross whose mood had been
low for some time, probably as a result of bullying. Eventually
his parents persuaded him to see his GP, making the appointment on his behalf and accompanying him to the surgery.
However, Ross wanted to consult with the doctor by himself,
and his parents, respecting his nascent autonomy, stayed in
the waiting room.

During the consultation it became clear that Ross was
severely depressed, and he confessed to the doctor something

that no one, not even his parents, knew: he had recently tried to commit suicide. The GP recognised that the attempt had been serious – no mere 'cry for help' – and made an urgent referral to the child and adolescent mental health service (CAMHS). Contact should have been made the following day but a transcription error meant the wrong mobile number was given, and Ross never received the promised call. A computer-generated letter was sent out instead, which Ross subsequently opened, giving details of an appointment. Ross never attended, though. Before the appointment date he made a further suicide attempt, and this time his body was found hanging in his bedroom by his mother.

One focus at the inquest was the decision by Ross's GP not to breach Ross's confidentiality and inform his parents of the depth of his depression and his suicide risk. Had they been made aware, his parents said, they would have ensured someone was with him constantly. They were also ignorant of the details of the proposed CAMHS involvement, so had no idea that a phone contact had failed. When Ross's CAMHS appointment letter was looked at in the cold light of events, it was seen to be formal and stark and off-putting – a style parents would be familiar with, but inappropriate for an emotionally vulnerable youth.

Lessons have been learned about reducing the potential for errors in the urgent referral process, and about designing more adolescent-friendly stationery and letter content. Many people will also have sympathy with Ross's parents' impassioned plea that it should be made mandatory for a 16 or 17-year-old's parents to be informed in these cases, irrespective of the child's wish for confidentiality. They believe an adolescent with significant depression is a special case (akin

to the consent-refuser described above) in which only quali-
fied autonomy is appropriate. Set against this is the fact that
mental health issues affect 10-15% of children and adolescents,
and in many cases (though not in Ross's) family dysfunction, sometimes even abuse, is the underlying problem – a
problem, furthermore, that might only become disclosed with
time and trust. To require doctors to breach confidentiality
in those circumstances could have its own equally disastrous
consequences.

WHAT YOU EAT

W E'VE RECENTLY HAD a public spat between two organisations holding opposing views as to what we should be eating. In the blue corner, Public Health England (PHE), the body responsible for promoting the nation's health. In the red, a newly formed, not-for-profit group of doctors, nutritionists, and fitness enthusiasts, all of whom believe that official advice is plain wrong. They have styled themselves the Public Health Collaboration (PHC). To avoid abject confusion, we'll refer to PHE as the establishment, and PHC as the mavericks.

The establishment's guidelines were updated recently with publication of the revised 'Eatwell Guide'. The mavericks launched a counterattack a couple of months later with their own report, less snappily but more prescriptively titled, 'Eat Fat, Cut the Carbs and Avoid Snacking To Reverse Obesity and Type 2 Diabetes'. What followed was the academic equivalent of a punch-up. The establishment wheeled out numerous senior figures to cast doubt on the mavericks' methodological credentials, and to describe their proposals variously as misleading, irresponsible, and quite possibly fatal. For their part, the mavericks alleged conspiracy between the establishment and the food industry in pursuit of corporate profit.

The row centred on two putative villains of the nutritional world: saturated fat, and carbohydrates. These are our main sources of energy. The establishment view for the past 30 years has been that saturated fat is Bad, because of a supposed link to heart disease. As such, it must be kept to a minimum. Instead, the energy content of our diet should come principally from starchy carbohydrates (bread, pasta, rice, potatoes).

The mavericks argue that the evidence implicating fat in the development of heart disease is now discredited. Further, they believe that the establishment's low-fat high-carb diet is responsible for the epidemic of obesity and type 2 diabetes currently sweeping the UK. In essence, carbohydrate (in refined or processed form) provokes the biggest surges of insulin, and insulin promotes the formation and retention of body fat. The more our energy intake is derived from refined carbohydrate, the more we put on weight and struggle to lose it. Interestingly, this tendency may not be universal. Some genetic make-ups – which dispose to the 'insulin resistance' behind type 2 diabetes – may be particularly maladapted to a high-carbohydrate diet.

As with many dichotomies, there is some truth on either side, and neither tells the whole story. One way to understand the alarming rise in obesity and diabetes may be a 'time travel' documentary, in which a typical 2018 family lands back in the mid-1970s. The people they meet would, on the whole, look strikingly slimmer. The shops would also appear exceedingly dull – lots of ingredients but very few ready meals, no 'low fat' products stuffed full of sugar, no chicanes of confectionary-laden shelves to navigate on the way to the tills.

The children would feel short-changed. A standard chocolate bar would resemble a 'fun size' version today. Adults would be dismayed by the limited range and relative expense of the alcohol available. They may console themselves with a trip to the pub for a slap-up lunch, only to complain loudly about the measly size of the portions.

Present-day mavericks watching the documentary would be heartened by the fat being consumed: meat for most meals, dripping-on-toast for Sunday tea, gold-top milk (less that siphoned off by enterprising birds). Establishment-types would crow at the sugar being ladled on to cereals, and the bread to fill hungry voids. Both would be alarmed at the paucity of fruit, though perhaps not veg, and struck by the sight of children and parents walking to school, the station, the shops. And the kids roaming in their free-time, covering miles in exploration and play.

Energy-rich foods have always been with us, but now we're bombarded. And burning this fuel is no longer an everyday feature of our lives. Carbohydrate, fat; it doesn't really matter. Eat less and do more. It's as simple – and as complicated – as that.

HARD RATIONS

In 2017, after nearly a decade of austerity underfunding, a snap general election that started out being dominated by Britain's proposed withdrawal from the European Union, gradually shifted focus into the parlous state of public services, not least the NHS.

P EOPLE SUFFERING FROM a range of health problems are experiencing the hard reality of the Conservatives' austerity NHS. Money has been getting progressively tighter for several years and, to put it bluntly, we're well past the point where we can do everything we used to do.

Nationally, the provision of gluten-free foods on prescription for people with coeliac disease is ceasing. Hayfever sufferers are to be expected to buy their treatments over-the-counter; likewise those needing paracetamol or ibuprofen for flu or muscular pains. This won't matter to working adults on a decent wage: the NHS prescription charge means it's already cheaper to purchase these kinds of things directly. But for those entitled to free prescriptions – either by virtue of age or low income – this will represent yet another drain on already stretched household budgets.

Similar rationing is happening with operations. Cataract removal, hernia repair, varicose vein treatment, bunion excision, together with a whole host of less common surgical procedures, are now subject to a highly bureaucratic process to obtain 'prior funding approval'. Already hard-pressed GPs are faced with lengthy forms to complete, and accompanying letters to be written, all to plead for treatments that used to be done routinely on the strength of a simple referral. The sheer weight of administration is intentional: put hurdles in the way, and many people will decide they simply haven't the energy to make the jump. Even for patients whose doctors do manage to scale the paperwork mountain, only those with the most severe conditions will get their treatment approved by the funding committee.

We discussed these developments at our local Clinical Commissioning Group recently. This is the forum where GPs in the locality get together to plan healthcare for our population. Most accepted the new reality with the weary resignation of a profession feeling powerless in the face of the irresistible forces grinding it down.

There were some glimmers of spirit, though. One of my colleagues, responding to a gloomy presentation from our chairman on the state of our finances, posed the question: rather than restricting services, can't we look at creative ways to raise more funds instead? She wondered about applying to charitable foundations, or partnering with commercial concerns. Her ideas were dismissed by the CCG leadership.

It set me thinking. Looking round a cathedral nowadays, one invariably finds a large, glass-domed receptacle in the entrance, with signage explaining how much it costs to maintain the building, and inviting visitors to make a donation. When booking for the theatre or various other attractions, I've become used to being asked to make a voluntary contribution over and above the cost of the ticket. And, like most parents, it's become a matter of course for my children's schools to seek parental help in meeting the cost of educational trips or equipment.

I raised my hand and sketched my off-the-cuff vision. How about a slip, given out with every NHS prescription, inviting additional voluntary contributions? And what about a big glass-domed receptacle in the A&E waiting room, with a sign explaining how much it costs to keep the hospital running each year, and inviting people, if they've enjoyed their visit, to make a donation?

The idea caused a few wry chuckles round the room. I fancied I could see the colour draining out of our CCG chairman's face, as he imagined being peremptorily summoned by the Department of Health to discuss the politically unacceptable developments in the health service in our area. Like my colleague's, my proposal got short shrift.

Brexit is important, but arguably it is drowning out other vital issues in this snap election. The NHS is inexorably becoming a minimum safety net for the have-nots, while the haves vote with their feet and utilise their greater resources to secure better provision privately. And what's true in health is also true in education, and social care. There is precious little time for opposition parties to get the parlous state of our public services firmly up the election agenda. Five more years of Tory austerity (at least) simply doesn't bear thinking about.

BORDER GUARDS

It isn't just chronic underfunding fuelling the NHS crisis:
Martini healthcare has to take its share of the blame.

THE RED CROSS came in for some stick recently when it warned that English hospitals are in state of 'humanitarian crisis'. Whatever one thinks of this description – provoked by the sight of innumerable sick patients languishing on trolleys in A&E corridors, or even bedded down on pushed-together chairs – it's worth pursuing the analogy a little.

Take Prime Minister Theresa May's pronouncement that the NHS's ills will be solved by pressuring GP surgeries to open 8 till 8, seven days a week. This was about as insightful as asserting that the refugee crisis in Europe will be addressed by extending the working hours of border guards. We need to consider the forces driving the migration (why patients are flooding into hospitals) and how we assess asylum claims (how we sort out who actually needs hospital care).

There are two drivers to the migration. The first concerns the ever-growing number of frail, usually elderly people with chronic health problems in our communities. Many of them only manage to live at home thanks to threadbare social support. Even with optimal medical treatment, exacerbations in their long-term health conditions happen with grinding regularity, with sudden and dramatic increases in care needs. There simply aren't enough resources at the moment to upgrade support to look after these patients safely at home. So in to hospital they go. And in hospital they stay, until they either no longer require enhanced community care, or it can somehow be squeezed out of an already overstretched system.

The solution to this, to return to the Red Cross analogy, is to establish high-quality camps closer to refugees' countries of origin. We need to fund flexible, responsive community care – and some 'hospital at home' treatments like IV antibiotics and fluids – to get people through short-term exacerbations without admitting them, and to enable earlier discharge from district generals if they do go in. Increasing 'cottage hospital' provision, which represents lower tech, less expensive inter-mediate-level care, would also be helpful. All this will take lots of investment, and lots of additional staff. Lots. Try running a proximate refugee camp on a shoestring and you'll soon discover how little it will do to stem the tide heading for the nearest border.

The other driver of the migration is the cultural shift to Martini-style health care – any time, any place, anywhere. We seem hellbent as a society on cramming our lives as full as possible, so we want supermarkets open at midnight, pizzas delivered at 4am, and advice about little Johnny's rash some-where in between. This began decades ago, but the creation of NHS111, which was supposed to meet this demand, has only aggravated matters. It was deemed too expensive to have sufficient numbers of clinicians available 24/7 to deal with the huge call volumes, so initial contacts are dealt with by non-clinicians operating a computer algorithm. The system is highly risk-adverse, and generates large numbers of 999 calls, or advice to attend A&E immediately, for problems that an ex-perienced GP would resolve without involving a hospital at all.

It is this Martini aspect that underlies Theresa May's prescription for longer opening hours in our surgeries. The problem is, there is a crisis in GP recruitment and retention already, and the harder you flog the existing workforce, the more will vote with their feet, and the fewer will be attracted to enter general practice in the first place. Remember that 2015 Tory manifesto commitment to find an extra 5,000 GPs from somewhere by 2020? No, neither do they.

It's probably impossible to reverse the culture of Martini healthcare, so we have to come up with a system that has experienced clinicians managing the first point of contact, keeping people well away from the border who don't need to go to a hospital. This will take lots of investment, and lots of additional staff. Lots. Sound familiar?

The bottom line is, we're getting the health and social care we currently pay for. It's an oft-quoted statistic: our percentage of GDP spent on health is among the lowest in the developed world. But higher public spending is anathema to the current government. The crisis is going to run on for a while yet.

IN HOURS

BROKEN HEART SYNDROME

MEDICINE HAS SOME fantastic diagnostic labels. My favourite is exploding head syndrome. Not as messy as it sounds, EHS is an example of a hypnagogic experience - phenomena that occur during the brain's transition from wakefulness to sleep. Most people will be familiar with the commonest of these - an abrupt sensation of falling. In EHS, the slumberer is jerked awake by a deafening bang emanating from inside their skull. It's over in a flash, leaving the person alarmed but otherwise unharmed - although doctors unfamiliar with the phenomenon may perform urgent scans and lumbar punctures, confusing EHS with a 'thunderclap headache', an ominous symptom that warns of an impending brain haemorrhage.

Pott's puffy tumour, by contrast, sounds almost cuddly, the sort of thing that might befall a character in a children's book. It presents with a large, boggy swelling over the forehead, caused by an abscess in and around the frontal bone of the skull. Teenagers are most prone, the puffy tumour forming as a result of infection spreading from the sinuses; if untreated it causes life-threatening brain complications. Puffy tumours became uncommon following the development of antibiotics in the mid-20th century, but have staged something of a comeback in recent decades due to an association with snorting cocaine.

Perhaps the most poignant label is that which Maria

encountered. She presented as an emergency with pains in her chest and shortness of breath. As a female non-smoker in her late forties, Maria was unlikely to have heart disease, and these symptoms occur frequently with panic attacks and anxiety. Maria, I knew, had been under enormous strain. Her beloved father had died a couple of months earlier, and once the contents of his will were made known, a full-blown war had erupted within the family. Bitter arguments over inheritance had reignited emotional traumas from the past: fault lines had reopened, siblings were no longer speaking, and legal action was being mooted.

Yet although Maria's symptoms sounded to be stress-related, my examination forced a rethink. No amount of emotional upheaval, I reasoned, could account for the abnormal sounds coming from her heart, nor the fluid I could detect on her lungs. An ECG returned a grossly abnormal trace: it seemed Maria was indeed having a heart attack. I sent her to hospital in a blue-light ambulance.

The cardiologists took her straight to angiography, where dye injected into the blood stream delineates the arteries supplying the heart muscle with oxygen. To everyone's surprise, there was no blockage, which is what one would normally see with a heart attack. Instead, Maria's heart itself had assumed a grotesquely abnormal shape. The apex of the main pumping chamber, the left ventricle, had blown up like a balloon, its usually thick muscular walls stretched thin and barely contracting.

A diagnosis of takotsubo cardiomyopathy was made. This is a strange condition, usually precipitated by grief or other profound emotional shocks. The heart muscle seems somehow to become stunned, causing it to malfunction and fail. The mechanism is not currently understood, but it may be the result of an aberrant reaction to high levels of adrenaline.

The name originates in Japan, where the condition was first documented in 1990. It can be fatal, but if, like Maria, the patient survives the initial phase, complete recovery occurs within a couple of months.

It's a classic example of medical technology belatedly catching up with folk wisdom. It has long been known that a severe emotional shock can cause sudden death, but only with the advent of sophisticated imaging techniques can we now see what is actually happening to the heart. 'Tako tsubo' means 'octopus pot'; the bizarre shape of the failing heart is reminiscent of a traditional Japanese fisherman's trap. But I prefer the anglicised version, 'broken heart syndrome', which Maria's bereavement and family trauma had precipitated. A few months later she is off medication, but the emotional wounds will take far longer to heal.

A REAL HEADACHE

CHERYL PRESENTED WITH three months of daily headaches. She'd tried various combinations of over-the-counter painkillers, none of which had made the blindest bit of difference. It was getting ridiculous, she couldn't go on like this, it was affecting every aspect of her life, she had to have some help. As I listened to her opening remarks it was clear she'd been shouldering mounting anxiety and, now she'd finally decided to consult a doctor, it all came tumbling out in a great rush of words.

This is a common scenario in general practice; one, furthermore, in which the subtitles to the consultation reel out a predictable script. Underlying the patient's discourse is the dread that they have something sinister – a brain tumour – but they hardly dare speak the concern for fear that it may, in fact, come true. For the doctor, knowing that brain tumours rarely present with isolated headaches, the task is two-fold: to draw the anxieties out into the open so they can be addressed; and to establish the true nature of the problem, which is usually something more prosaic.

In Cheryl's case, it proved relatively easy to get to the nub of her concerns. She readily admitted that not one but two relatives had suffered from brain tumours in the past. She'd been living with these headaches, hoping they would pass off, but as the weeks had turned to months she had developed the near-certainty that she was following in the footsteps of her unfortunate kin.

Now her concerns were aired, I set about trying to establish the cause. The vast majority of headache encountered in primary care is one of two sorts: tension headache or migraine. Tension headaches affect people at times of turmoil. Many of us sink our stresses in the muscles of our neck and shoulders, which gives rise to the pervasive pain of tension headache. A vicious circle ensues, with growing fear as to the possibility of cancer aggravating the original stresses and compounding the physical symptoms. Cheryl was adamant, though: everything in her twenty-one-year-old life was fine. Good job, happy relationships, no money worries. Nothing that would set in train a spiral of tension headache.

I asked about features of migraine. There is usually a family history – there is a genetic basis to the complaint – but no one in Cheryl's family was a diagnosed migraineur. And migraines come with added 'colour'. This might be vomiting, or transient paralysis of a limb, or a disturbance in vision – sometimes jagged lines in the visual field (fortification spectra), sometimes reversible loss of sight in one eye. Cheryl had none of these, but she did volunteer that for the past few weeks her vision had been very blurred when she woke, slowly clarifying as the morning wore on.

This is not a migrainous phenomenon, and it piqued my attention. I asked more about the pattern of the headaches. They never woke her from sleep, she told me, but they were at their worst first thing, easing somewhat as the morning went on. Now I mentioned it, she had noticed the pain worsening were she to sneeze, or to lean down to pick something up. These features suggest aggravation by activities that cause a rise in the pressure in the head. Sinus congestion would be the commonest explanation, but Cheryl had no catarrhal symptoms.

Measurement of her height and weight put her body mass index (BMI) over 40. A healthy BMI lies between 18 – 25; anything over 35 is morbid obesity. Her blood pressure was normal, but examination of the back of her eye revealed papilloedema – blurring of the margins of the optic disc. The optic disc is the root of the nerve that takes the fibres from the retina back into the brain. Swelling of the disc indicates that the fluid around the brain is under high pressure – intracranial hypertension.

Intracranial hypertension is never an innocent finding and can indeed be a consequence of a brain tumour. I started to share some of Cheryl's anxiety, but her age and her BMI pointed to a more perplexing cause. Idiopathic intracranial hypertension (IIH) was a mere footnote in the textbooks when I trained, but it is becoming ever more common with the obesity epidemic. And while it used to be considered benign, we now appreciate that, untreated, it can cause permanent damage to vision.

IIH affects young women with substantially raised BMIs. The term idiopathic means 'no one knows the cause'. The mechanisms are still obscure, but some interaction between morbid obesity and the female hormonal milieu results in chronically elevated pressure in the fluid around the brain and spinal cord (cerebrospinal fluid, or CSF) resulting in just the pattern of headaches Cheryl was experiencing and, in more advanced cases, swelling of the optic disc affecting eyesight.

I referred her urgently to a neurologist. A brain scan thankfully ruled out any tumour, and a lumbar puncture – inserting a needle into the space around the spinal cord – confirmed, and allowed relief of, the elevated CSF pressure. Acetazolamide, a medication that slows production of CSF, helps, but the only permanent resolution is with weight loss, which will take many months. Once Cheryl attains a more normal BMI, the obscure factors that are driving the rise in her CSF pressure will recede, curing the headaches and improving her health in numerous other ways besides.

STRESS TEST

ON THE FACE of it, Helen's employers were looking after her well: head of HR, her package of benefits included an annual health screen, presumably to head off any incipient problems that might affect her ability to render the company good service. She'd attended one recently, expecting to be assured she was fighting fit. Instead, she'd been told it looked like she had ischaemic heart disease, and had been urged to see her GP.

She was keeping calm, but was understandably disconcerted. I was puzzled. In her mid-forties, a never-smoker, with blameless blood pressure, a healthy weight, a moderately active lifestyle, and an unremarkable family history, it was difficult to conceive of a candidate less likely to develop angina, or be struck down by a heart attack.

The problem was, as part of her screening, she'd undergone a stress test. This involved her being connected to an ECG – which records electrical activity in the heart – and then being put through progressively more strenuous exercise on a treadmill. Some way into the test, Helen's ECG had developed changes – known as ST depression – that are associated with the heart becoming starved of oxygen (ischaemia). Ischaemia occurs when an artery supplying the heart muscle is critically narrowed by fatty deposits known as atheroma.

It's usually accompanied by chest pain or tightness. Helen assured me she'd felt nothing. And, no, she never experienced such things, even when running or doing aerobics. By now I was convinced she was in danger of becoming a victim of the health-screening industry.

Stress tests, like all medical investigations, generate false positive results. Estimates vary, but it probably happens in about 1 in 10. That's OK if you're performing the stress test to make a diagnosis. Say you have ten patients all complaining of chest pain; a good proportion – let's say 50% – will have underlying ischaemic heart disease. When you test all ten, five will therefore generate a true positive result, but a sixth will be a false positive. So, 5 out of every 6 positives reflect genuine heart trouble, meaning a positive result has an 85% chance of being 'right'. Not perfect, but useful when deciding who to investigate further.

However, look what happens if you use the same test to screen ten healthy people like Helen, none of who actually has anything wrong. You'll get one positive result, but it will be false: the test is wrong 100% of the time. Even if one of the ten symptomless people does in fact have unsuspected heart disease (and that's a big if), you'll end up with two positives, only one of which is true – so a positive result has only a 50% chance of being 'right'. You might as well flip a coin. To cap it all, false positives are very common in pre-menopausal women like Helen, because oestrogen disposes towards benign ST depression when exercising.

Helen wasn't to know any of this. From her perspective, she'd been to a reputable medical company, who'd wired her up to some impressive gadgetry that had raised serious concerns about her health. Even once I'd explained the ins and outs, a part of her mind was still thinking, 'Yes, but. What if my result was actually true?' There are invasive investigations that could settle the question definitively, but they involve exposure to radiation or risk of stroke.

There was no way out of the conundrum created by the unethical use of a diagnostic test for screening. The private screening industry is essentially unregulated, and causes substantial worry – and sometimes consequent physical harm – all in the pursuit of profit. The same issues apply to its misuse of other diagnostic tests such as CT and MRI scans. And it's the NHS that's left picking up the pieces when inevitable false positives turn up.

In time, Helen regained the health-confidence that her brush with the private screening industry had undermined. It will be interesting to see whether she politely declines her next invitation to be screened – or, indeed, whether her employers allow her to do so.

VIDEO STAR

ONE OF THE most useful tools I have as a GP trainer is my video camera. Periodically, and always with patients' permission, I place it in the corner of my registrar's room. We then look through their consultations together during a tutorial.

There's nothing quite like watching oneself at work to spur development. One of my trainees – a lovely guy called Nick – was appalled to find that he wheeled his chair closer and closer to the patient as he narrowed down the diagnosis with a series of questions. It was entirely unconscious, but somewhat intimidating, and he never repeated it once he'd seen the recording. Whether it's spending half the consultation staring at the computer screen, or slipping into baffling technospeak, or parroting 'OK' after every comment a patient makes, we all have unhelpful mannerisms of which we are blithely unaware until observing ourselves in action.

Videos are a great way of understanding how patients communicate, too. Another registrar, Anthony, had spent several years as a rheumatologist before switching to general practice, so when consulted by Yvette he felt on familiar ground. She began by saying she thought she had carpal tunnel syndrome (CTS) – a constellation of pain, numbness, and sometimes muscle weakness caused by a nerve getting trapped in a confined space – the carpal tunnel – at the wrist.

Anthony confirmed the diagnosis with some clinical tests,

then went on to establish the impact it was having on Yvette's life. Her sleep was disturbed every night, and she was no longer able to pick up and carry her young children. Her desperation for a swift cure came across loud and clear.

The consultation then ran into difficulty. There are three things that can help CTS: wrist splints, steroid injections, and surgery to release the nerve. Splints are usually the preferred first option because they carry no risk of complications, and are inexpensive to the NHS. We watched as Anthony tried to explain this. Yvette kept raising objections, and even though Anthony did his best to address her concerns, it was clear she remained unconvinced.

The problem for Anthony, as for many doctors, is that much medical training still reflects an era when patients relied heavily on professionals for health information. Today, most people will have consulted extensively with Dr Google before presenting to their GP. Sometimes this will have stoked unfounded fears – pretty much any symptom just might be an indication of cancer – and our task then is to put things in proper context. But frequently, as with Yvette, patients have not only worked out what is wrong, they also have clear ideas what to do about it.

We played the video through again, and I highlighted the numerous subtle cues Yvette had offered. Like many patients, she was reticent about stating outright what she wanted, but the information was there in what she did and didn't say, and in how she responded to Anthony's suggestions. By the time we'd finished analysing their exchanges, Anthony could see Yvette had already decided against splints as being too cumbersome and taking too long to work. For her, a steroid injection was the quickest and surest way to obtain relief.

Competing considerations must be weighed in any 'shared' decision between a doctor and patient. Autonomy - the ability for a patient to determine their own care - is of prime importance, but it isn't unrestricted. The balance between doing good and doing harm, about which doctors sometimes have a far clearer appreciation, has to be factored in. Then there are questions of equity and fairness - within a finite NHS budget, doctors have a duty to prioritise the most cost-effective treatments. Going straight for surgery wouldn't have been right for the NHS or for Yvette - nor did she want it - but a steroid injection is both low cost and low risk, and Anthony could see he'd missed the chance to maximise her autonomy. The lessons he learned from the video had a powerful impact on him, and from that day on he became much more adept at achieving truly shared decisions with his patients.

CATAPLEXY

BEN WAS NODDING off at the drop of a hat: during meals, in the cinema, even partway through teaching a class. Review of his lifestyle failed to unearth an inner party animal that might be held responsible. Blood tests ruled out under-active thyroid or diabetes. But his score on the Epworth Sleepiness Scale was impressively dire: something was wrong.

The commonest explanation would be obstructive sleep apnoea (OSA), where heavy snoring actually halts breathing repeatedly throughout the night. The resulting periods of low blood oxygen cause profound fatigue the following day, though patients think they've slept well. But OSA principally affects the obese. Ben wasn't exactly svelte – in fact, he also complained that he was putting on weight inexplicably – but his collar size was still below the 17-inch threshold associated with OSA.

The only way to tell for sure, though, would be a sleep study. Ben spent a night at the local sleep unit, wired up to all manner of monitoring equipment. There was no evidence of apnoea attacks, which ruled out OSA. The consultant there raised the possibility of a condition called narcolepsy. This affects just 1 in 2,500 people, and arises when brain cells producing a substance called hypocretin die off. Hypocretin plays a crucial role in regulating the sleep-wake cycle.

A different sort of study is needed to diagnose narcolepsy – a multiple sleep latency test (MSLT). This measures how swiftly someone falls asleep when napping during the day, and also charts what type of sleep they enter. People with narcolepsy zonk out at the click of a finger, and typically move straight into rapid-eye-movement (REM) sleep. Once again Ben was hooked up to the monitors. However, on no occasion did he demonstrate the characteristic immediate-REM pattern.

The consultant discharged him saying narcolepsy was excluded, and recommending I refer him to an endocrinologist in case the fatigue and weight gain indicated some obscure hormonal problem. Ben came in to discuss things, and at one point he mentioned odd episodes where his legs would buckle beneath him if he was laughing, or if he'd been surprised by something.

It rang a bell. 'Did you mention that to the consultant?'

'Definitely,' he said. 'I remember telling him I'd collapsed at crazy golf.'

I phoned the sleep specialist the next day. Like me, he immediately recognised that Ben was describing a second disorder, cataplexy, where a sudden emotional jolt causes a reflex loss of muscle tone in the limbs. And cataplexy, too, is related to low hypocretin levels – it often goes hand in hand with narcolepsy.

'We'd better get him back up,' the consultant said.

This time he performed a lumbar puncture – tapping fluid from around the spinal cord – and sent it for hypocretin assay. Sure enough, Ben's levels were very low. A rare instance of a narcolepsy sufferer who doesn't nap straight into REM sleep.

The case reminded me of several important lessons. First, all tests can produce false results: Ben's consultant had interpreted the MSLT as excluding narcolepsy, and his confidence in the result had led him to miss a textbook description of cataplexy. Secondly, we should remain healthily sceptical about other doctors' opinions: if I'd have accepted the consultant's verdict at face value, Ben might still be undiagnosed. Thirdly, we should never be too proud to change our mind: as soon as the consultant realised his thinking had gone astray, he acted to put matters right.

And finally, knowledge is never complete. What neither the consultant nor I were aware of was that hypocretin has recently been linked to body mass regulation. High levels stimulate 'brown fat' tissue, which burns off rather than stores calories; conversely, lower levels are associated with more ready weight gain. Ben had been describing a clue neither of us had appreciated.

Fascinatingly, hypocretin might hold the key as to why some of us find it easier to stay slim than others. And there is the intriguing possibility that hypocretin augmentation might represent a future treatment for obesity. Meanwhile, Ben's narcolepsy has responded to drug therapy, and he is managing to keep himself awake once again.

TOP OF THE EAR DISEASE

A FEW YEARS ago, a mum brought her young sons along with crops of itchy blisters along the tops of their ears. I'd never seen anything like it. Both boys were otherwise well, and neither had a single blemish elsewhere.

I reasoned it must be an allergy, but there was no new hair product that might have set it off, and neither of them wore glasses or hats or sweatbands; nothing that could have brought a chemical into contact with their ears.

I considered a virus. Many show a predilection for certain areas of skin – Hand, Foot and Mouth Disease causes spots in just those three locations. However, Top of the Ear Disease seemed unlikely. I was stumped. But, whatever the cause, it looked like some steroid cream to damp down the inflammation would help.

The following week, Annie, one of the other GPs, caught me at coffee time.

'I saw those boys,' she said. There was amusement in her eyes. 'It's juvenile spring eruption.'

She filled me in. JSE is one of medicine's curios. As the name implies, it's a seasonal phenomenon, where the first spell of spring sunshine provokes an itchy, blistering rash confined to the tops of the ears. Intriguingly, it occurs in sporadic outbreaks, thought to be because a combination of strong sunlight and particularly cold air is required. Boys are more commonly affected, presumably because of short-back-and-sides. And people grow out of it during their teens, hence the specific age-group.

JSE is treated by steroid cream – so at least I'd got that right – and avoidance of strong sunlight, which Annie had been able to advise the boys' mum about when they came for review.

Much diagnosis is pattern-recognition. If, like Annie, I'd encountered JSE before, I would have known instantly what I was dealing with. Because I hadn't, I'd been left figuring it out from first principles. I'd deduced the basics – an external agent causing an inflammatory reaction – but I was kicking myself for not considering sunlight. I've seen many UV reactions, most commonly when a medication has sensitised the skin, but they have a tell-tale distribution, affecting all sun-exposed areas. In JSE, the chill air sensitises the peripheral ears alone.

The case came to mind recently, when Health Secretary Jeremy Hunt – admitting that NHS111 is woefully short of clinician-involvement – advised parents to Google their children's rashes instead. This caused an outcry among doctors, concerned that parents might waste crucial time trying to work out if the non-blanching rash really was life-threatening meningococcal sepsis. But I wondered whether Hunt's approach might be useful for a benign, esoteric condition like JSE.

Searching 'itchy rash ears' did throw up a few medical articles with JSE mentioned in the small print, but they weren't much help to the uninitiated. Much more use were the long threads about JSE on three different 'Mumsnet'-type sites. Post after post expressed delight at having encountered others with the same puzzling problem. Astutely, the preponderance of boys was remarked on by several contributors, and some, whose children had been affected in previous years, made the seasonal connection. Pollen was considered as a cause, logical given common knowledge of another seasonal condition, hayfever. Posts from 2010 speculated whether the Icelandic volcanic ash cloud might be responsible – a lovely illustration of our tendency to link unusual events causally.

Posts reporting medical consultations showed I was far from the only doctor never to have encountered JSE. On every thread, though, someone eventually took their child to see an Annie, and JSE was diagnosed. Once it was, it made perfect sense to everyone, and the threads closed in a welter of well-I-never posts.

No one made the diagnosis solely from their own internet research; doctors aren't entirely redundant. But medicine is such a vast field, we medics have to keep learning lifelong. I haven't seen another JSE case since those boys, but every springtime I wonder whether this will be my year to shine.

DNAR

MARTINA WAS SEVENTY-EIGHT when I first met her. She had recently undergone a major operation for thyroid cancer, and had moved to be near her son. She was on a bewildering array of medications – for blood pressure, arthritis, diabetes, osteoporosis, plus three different heart conditions. Over a series of consultations I gradually got to grips with her medical history. I also got to know her. Her voice had been rendered permanently gravelly by the surgery. It suited her understated, dry humour.

Martina wanted to be on as few drugs as possible, so I drew up a 'hit list' of the ones she would be least likely to miss. We managed to trim four, but in discontinuing the fifth we provoked a spectacular upset in the delicate balance with her heart. We agreed we had probably got rid of all that we reasonably could.

A couple of years later she developed neck pain that turned out to be from cancer metastases in her spine. She accepted the news with equanimity, and was happy to engage in 'advance care planning' – establishing her attitudes to future care in the face of a terminal diagnosis. She had no hesitation in deciding against cardiopulmonary resuscitation (CPR) in the event of a natural death.

Over the next year Martina's cancer deposits showed little progression. In fact, it was her ailing heart that was causing increasing problems – fatigue, breathlessness, and disturbed sleep. With that and her worsening arthritis, she was no longer able to get out of the house. I began to visit her at home. She remained mentally sparky, and I enjoyed our conversations, but it was sad to witness her physical decline.

Then one weekend, she suffered a heart attack. Alone and in pain she dialled 999, and shortly after opening the door to the paramedics she collapsed and died. There should have been a Do Not Attempt Resuscitation (DNAR) flag on her ambulance service records, but it had failed to migrate during a system change. She had a paper DNAR notice stuck to the door of her fridge; the paramedics never saw it. They launched straight into CPR and, amazingly, Martina become one of the 10% of patients to be successfully brought back from an out-of-hospital cardiac arrest.

I visited her after her subsequent discharge. I asked how she felt about having been resuscitated against her wishes. She was sitting across from me in her lounge, bathed in the spring sunlight streaming through her window. She gave me a wry smile, gesticulated at the wonderful weather outside – weather she could enjoy but only through glass – and confessed that she really didn't know.

Over the ensuing couple of months her heart failure progressed relentlessly. Despite fine-tuning her medication, her legs became permanently swollen and her breathing was laboured with the slightest activity. There were a couple of crisis admissions during which the hospital patched up exacerbations, then it was back home for more of the same.

I felt she must surely have come to rue that unwanted resuscitation, so depressing was this subsequent downward spiral. But in fact, her brush with death seemed to have given her a renewed joy in life, despite the hardships. She even spoke of reversing her previous DNAR decision, though she had come to no settled conclusion before the next emergency admission, from which she did not return.

The burgeoning number of frail elderly patients with multiple health problems has led to an NHS-wide push to expand advance care planning. In some ways this is good, preventing futile heroics being performed on people at the very end of life. But Martina's story illustrates how difficult it can be to imagine how we might truly feel about some hypothetical future state of health. It begs the question as to how valid these decisions may sometimes be. And it reinforces for me that, even when we professionals might judge someone's quality of life to have become extremely poor, to them it may still be something they relish. It can be incredibly hard for any of us to know when the time has come finally to let go.

NEW BOOKS FROM SALT

SAMUEL FISHER
The Chameleon (978-1-78463-124-6)

KERRY HADLEY-PRYCE
Gamble (978-1-78463-130-7)

BEE LEWIS
Liminal (978-1-78463-138-3)

VESNA MAIN
Temptation: A User's Guide (978-1-78463-128-4)

ALISON MOORE
Missing (978-1-78463-140-6)

S.J. NAUDÉ
The Third Reel (978-1-78463-150-5)

HANNAH VINCENT
The Weaning (978-1-78463-120-8)

This book has been typeset by
SALT PUBLISHING LIMITED
using Neacademia, a font designed by Sergei Egorov
for the Rosetta Type Foundry in the Czech Republic. It
is manufactured using Holmen Book Cream 70gsm, a
Forest Stewardship Council™ certified paper from the
Hallsta Paper Mill in Sweden. It was printed and bound
by Clays Limited in Bungay, Suffolk, Great Britain.

CROMER
GREAT BRITAIN
MMXVIII